Jump Off
the Mood Swing

Jump Off
the Mood Swing

*A Sane Woman's Guide to
Her Crazy Hormones*

Brendan McCarthy

Protea Life

Jump Off the Mood Swing: A Sane Woman's Guide to Her Crazy Hormones

Published by Protea Life

Copyright © 2018 by Dr. Brendan McCarthy

Protea Life
1949 West Ray Rd, Suite 10
Chandler, AZ 85224
Email: Publishing@ProteaLife.com

Publishing and editorial team:
Author Bridge Media, www.AuthorBridgeMedia.com
Project Manager and Editorial Director: Helen Chang
Editor: Jenny Shipley
Publishing Manager: Laurie Aranda
Publishing Coordinator: Iris Sasing
Cover Design: Paul Kimber

ISBN: 978-0-9996496-0-2 – softcover
       978-0-9996496-1-9 – hardcover
       978-0-9996496-2-6 – ebook

Ordering Information:
Quantity sales. Special discounts are available on quantity purchases by corporations, associations, and others. For details, contact the publisher at the address above.

Printed in United States of America.

DEDICATION

To my wife, Celeste—you are the greatest source of love and inspiration in my life.

To my children, Liam, Audrey, and Aedan—be bold in life.

And to my patients—thank you for your trust, your courage, and your faith.

ACKNOWLEDGMENTS

Thank you to Celeste, for helping me become who I've always wanted to be.

I would also like to thank Dr. Lily Siou (Chang Yi Hsiang), for setting the foundation; Dr. Paul Anderson, for teaching me how to think; Dr. Walter Crinnion, for teaching me how to learn; and Patrick Olwell, for showing me what is possible.

Thank you to Katherine MacKenett, Jenny Shipley, and the team at Author Bridge Media for helping find the words to share my vision.

And most of all, thank you to my patients. When I have given you health, you have given me purpose, and for that I am eternally grateful.

CONTENTS

INTRODUCTION

Two Voices

This is not right.

You probably recognize this thought. It comes from that voice in the back of your head—your inner nature—the *something* inside that's in touch with who you are. You hear it when you feel defeated by your own life: anxious, irritable, unable to sleep. You hear it when you're depressed. You sense it when you feel held back, not taking the risks you want to take, and not living your life to the fullest—when everything feels completely unhinged, and you don't know how to address it.

No, says the very quiet voice. *This is not right. I shouldn't feel this way.*

At the same time, everyone around you—society, your family, your friends, your doctors, *everyone*—tells you that you're supposed to experience these emotions. Since you were a little girl, you've been taught that this is "just the way it is." It has been drilled into you by everything from parents to TV shows: women are supposed to be cranky; women are anxious and irritable; it's natural for women to suffer from

PMS symptoms. These archetypes are constantly presented as normal.

So a second voice shows up in your head. A louder voice.

What am I complaining about? There's nothing wrong with me. Every other woman deals with this stuff. I just need to suck it up and deal with it too.

And for a long time, you do. You live with it. You suppress it. You compensate for it in so many other ways. You tune it out in order to achieve the things you need to achieve in life.

But it never really goes away. And that first voice is still there in the back of your head, saying, *This is not right . . .*

This is not right.

You want to be free of this anxiety—this feeling that something awful is always about to happen. You want to be free of irritability. You want to take that risk at your job and ask for a raise. You want to pursue spontaneous relationships, and you want to feel like going out to do something fun again.

You want to feel sane and at peace in your own skin. And that first voice is telling you, *There is a solution. You can get through this.*

But is there? And can you?

The Connection

Our inner nature doesn't lie. A path back to a manageable, fulfilling life exists.

That path begins with hormone balance.

Your whole body is interconnected. Every part of it connects to another piece. Each piece touches and influences another part.

The two elements with the most intense, intimate relationship in a woman's body are hormones and emotions.

Your brain chemistry is intimately guided by your hormones. Because of this, having imbalanced hormones influences everything from your confidence, to your assertiveness, to your ability to take chances, to your sense of peace in life.

How likely is it that what you feel is linked in some way to a hormone imbalance?

According to countless studies, the odds are about 100 percent. It's incredibly rare to find a woman with completely balanced hormones. But the good news is that hormone imbalance can be corrected. It's not even difficult to do.

And when your hormones come back into balance, it's almost like jumping off a swing that has been dragging you back and forth—a mood swing, if you will.

You're no longer rattled by things. All of a sudden, you realize, "Wow, that doesn't drive me crazy like it used to. I didn't get angry." You don't feel uncomfortable anymore. Your period comes each month, and it doesn't affect you as negatively as before. You have the confidence to ask for that raise at work—and you get it. You feel like going and doing something that you normally wouldn't do, so you go and do it. Everything is different.

You're empowered. You're wicked strong. You are your best you. And—finally—you have your life back.

The Cost of Tuning Out

At this point, I can guess your thoughts.

How do you know all this? You're a guy.

And you're right. I am a guy. There isn't much to us men. Biologically, we're pretty simple creatures. But women?

You women are *amazing*.

I've worked with some very empowered and strong women over the years. You're brilliant. You can tune out a profound amount of stress in your life to achieve what you need to achieve. Men can't do that the way you can.

But on the flip side of the coin, the stress takes a toll on you that most men can't imagine.

I know because I've heard your stories, over and over again—and I'm the kind of person who listens. I've built my life's work on listening first and then collaborating with patients to find solutions.

It's not that I was born with some rare talent for this. On the contrary, I owe the way I practice medicine to two people: my son Liam and a woman named Jenna Caruso.

My Path to Medicine

In the early 2000s, my first son, Liam, was born with a life-threatening disorder. And for weeks, no one could tell my wife and me what it was.

We saw every kind of doctor you can think of. All of them dismissed us with prescriptions that fell within their areas of specialization.

But nothing worked. And Liam was dying.

Finally, we met Dr. Mark Joseph, a nephrologist at Phoenix Children's Hospital, who admitted that he was in the dark. "I have no idea what is going on with this kid," he said. "Let me draw a big circle around the problem and run some tests. We'll keep looking until we've figured this out."

And that's exactly what he did. He listened to what was happening and then went after an answer using a systematic, targeted method. That was how we figured out that Liam had a rare genetic kidney disorder.

That was how we saved his life.

I was in medical school at the time, and the experience with Liam deeply affected me. That doctor who actually ran labs to figure out what was wrong with my son before treating him shifted my entire view of medicine.

That's the kind of doctor I want to be, I thought. *The kind who listens and draws a big circle around the problem until he figures it out.*

My chance to be that doctor showed up a couple of years later when a woman named Jenna Caruso walked into my clinic.

By then, I had graduated from medical school. At the time, I worked in a clinic dedicated to environmental toxicology. Jenna was one of those women who had a healthy lifestyle but felt terrible anyway—especially around her cycle.

The doctor I worked under focused on Jenna's mercury poisoning, which can cause emotional instability. But as her toxicology reports improved, her emotional symptoms did not. And my supervising physician gave me the freedom to investigate other possible causes.

I know her symptoms aren't due to mercury poisoning, I thought. *Her symptoms are cyclical, with her period, and mercury poisoning symptoms are constant. It's worth it to find a solution. She's worth my time and effort over the next couple of days to figure this out.*

So I started reading. I kept coming back to hormones, because Jenna's symptoms were strongly associated with her period. I ran a whole battery of tests and figured out exactly where Jenna was out of balance. Her progesterone was off, so I gave her a safe, natural supplement for it.

And Jenna got better. Fast.

Wow, I thought, as I watched Jenna take her life back. *This is powerful stuff.* I began researching even more about hormones to help more women like Jenna reclaim themselves and their lives. The more I saw these women transform, the more I knew I had found my calling.

And the rest is history.

An Experienced Hand

I've worked with thousands of women over the years to help them clear a path back to healthy, fulfilling lives.

I started my practice in 2002, and in 2004, I began teaching other physicians from around the country about hormone balance. I have trained more than one thousand doctors, and, since 2012, I've been the only physician in the United States who teaches hormone replacement therapy in this specific way.

But my biggest credential and best experiences are the patients who come to see me and keep coming back. I still see the very first patient I ever had. And those patients send their friends and family to see me, too.

What I do has never been about awards or degrees. It's always been about changing lives. To me, there's nothing more rewarding than that. I've had patients—women who were previously told they'd never have children—call me while I'm out driving to tell me they're pregnant because of the work we've done together. When that happens, I pull over to the side of the road and just cry with honest joy for them.

My work is more than a job for me; it's a calling. I believe in what I do because I've seen it transform literally thousands of lives. And I know it can transform yours as well.

Your Health Care Handbook

This book is designed to empower you. I wrote it to help you take your life back. It is a handbook for you to learn about your body and a tool to use in taking charge of your health.

You can bring this book into your doctor's office, point to cited research, and say, "This is what I believe I have going on." You will know what labs to request and the types of treatment to ask for. And if you need more information, I will provide further resources as well.

I want you to learn how to convert your doctor from being a sometimes-adversary into an all-the-time ally.

As you read this book, mark the passages that feel right for you. Use bookmarks, sticky notes, or highlighters—whatever you like, so you know specifically what you want to talk to your doctor about. Everything in each chapter may not apply to you. But I bet that at least one thing will.

Try to pay attention to places where you recognize yourself in what you're reading. If something lines up with your experience, make a note. You can discover, right now, more about what you need.

After you have read this book, you will be able to see and understand your personal path to empowered health care. And that will allow you to ask for the best solution for you.

You don't have to settle for anything less.

A Legacy of Wellness

Sometimes people ask me why I continued on this path after helping Jenna so long ago. Why am I, all these years later, still so inspired to serve women like her?

It's because of my mom.

My mom is a good person. She raised me with the help of my stepfather. But she really struggled with her hormones when I was growing up. I saw hormone imbalance rob my mother of her health and happiness. She suffered every month. And knowing what I know now, the hard truth is this: she suffered needlessly.

I do what I do to correct the system so that no child ever again has to watch his or her mother go through what mine went through. My mom could have had a better life. And her story doesn't need to happen to any woman in this day and age.

It doesn't have to be your story.

You don't have to feel anxious. You don't have to get edgy once a month. Imagine what it would feel like not to be depressed, in pain, or out of control of your own body and emotions. That can be you. If you have a hormone imbalance, it can be fixed. And the best part? Once you understand how to fix it, you can jump off the mood swing and *stay* off—forever.

I tell all of my patients, "I believe in you. I believe in who you really are. And the world is a better place with you here." You deserve to have an amazing life, and you deserve to be happy. Most of all, you deserve to *try* to make that happen.

It is worth it to find out what may be wrong inside your body and to fix it. You, yourself, are worth it.

Are you ready to move toward your most beautiful life?

Chapter 1

Overview

Finding Hope

"When I was twenty-one, a doctor at the Mayo Clinic told me I would never have children. I haven't had a period in ten years."

The woman sitting on the exam table in front of me was named Nicole. She was thirty-three years old. And glaring mistrust radiated from her like cold coming off a glacier.

Nicole had given up hope that she would ever be a mother. The only reason she had come to see me was because several of her friends were my patients, and they had urged her to give my clinic a try. But she made it very clear that this was my one chance.

I had to make it count.

So I proceeded carefully. I ordered lab work right away. Her estrogen was fine, but she had low progesterone and no testosterone whatsoever. Also, her prolactin level was extremely high—101, when it should have been 4. And that was strange because prolactin should be elevated only when a woman is nursing.

We started her on progesterone during the second half of her cycle, along with a short course of low-dose testosterone. We discontinued the testosterone when she started to make her own. We also encouraged her to change her diet.

A month later, she had her first period in ten years.

And a few months after that, I was driving home from work when Nicole called me. All of the ice from that first meeting had melted long ago. "I'm pregnant!" she told me, ecstatic.

I pulled to the side of the road and cried with her from sheer happiness. Over the course of several months, Nicole had gone from no hope to having everything she had always dreamed of. When she gave birth to a beautiful baby boy, she honored me by using my last name as his middle name.

By taking control of her hormones, Nicole took control of more than just her body. She took control of her life.

What Is Hormone Imbalance?

Your body is like a symphony.

Symphonies are composed of many different instruments playing different melodies, all weaving together to create beautiful music. For that arrangement to work, everything has to be in balance.

The same is true in your body. When the body's hormones are imbalanced, the symphony drifts out of tune.

Suddenly, dissonant chords start playing, and these can show up in many different ways. One woman's inharmonious body may make her feel anxious and depressed around her period. Another patient may have breast pain, heavy periods, or pain with intercourse. Yet another may experience insomnia, sugar cravings, and headaches.

All of these discordant symptoms can point to hormone imbalance.

But the good news is that the symphony doesn't have to stay out of tune. Hormones can be managed. Balance can be achieved. And when that happens, your symphony can play beautifully.

You don't have to experience pain every month. You don't need to suffer from cramps. You don't have to feel sick, crazy, and horrible, or like you must hide from society part of every month.

When your body finds its balance, it goes back to making beautiful music.

So what are hormones? What causes them to become out of balance? And how can you chart your personal course back to a life you love?

What Are Hormones?

Hormones are signals sent through the bloodstream from one part of the body to another.

Your hormones aren't limited to estrogen, progesterone, and testosterone. When we talk hormones, we're also talking thyroid. We're talking insulin. Think about someone who hasn't eaten, so his or her insulin is off—how crabby that person gets. Think about someone whose thyroid is too low and who is always tired, like Eeyore from *Winnie the Pooh*.

So many things play into hormone balance that entire books and journals have been written about it. At least two journals—*Hormones and Behavior* and *Frontiers in Neuroendocrinology*—publish hundreds of articles every year about hormones and brain chemistry, and that subject matter is their entire focus. Hormones are a big piece of the picture when it comes to our health.

So how do hormones work?

Hormones are generated through a series of complex reactions, starting from proteins, cholesterol, or minerals. These hormones travel through the bloodstream, serving as messages between organs and tissues. These signals regulate every aspect of your health, from your metabolism, fertility, and blood sugar levels to the aging process. Hormones directly affect metabolic and neurological activities such as digestion, perception, sleep, stress, growth and development, and mood.

Your nervous system works in this same way, sending signals from one part of the body to another, but it happens slightly differently. The endocrine system uses hormones, but the mind uses neurotransmitters to send a signal via the nerves. When hormones are released into circulation, however, they go throughout the whole body. And those hormones can affect your neurotransmitters.

All of these signals, whether sent through hormones or the nervous system, affect your body, mind, and mood. When hormones are off, they will create the physical symptoms you experience. This imbalance can throw off your neurotransmitters as well.

But what disrupts your hormone balance in the first place?

The Causes of Hormone Imbalance

Hormone imbalance may be caused by several factors, but the three most common triggers I see in American women are stress, diet, and the environment.

The sheer volume of stress in your life can throw your hormones out of balance. If you are under a lot of pressure, for example, your body will not ovulate. And if you do not ovulate, you will have too much estrogen and not enough progesterone. We'll talk about the consequences of this more in chapter 2.

Our modern diet can also contribute to this imbalance.

For example, for some women, dietary gluten can inappropriately increase prolactin.[1,2,3,4] As I mentioned earlier with Nicole, prolactin is a hormone that normally rises when a woman gives birth, causing her to lactate. It also inhibits ovulation, which again leads to low progesterone.

Your environment also affects your hormones. This is true for both women and men. In my entire career, I've seen only three men with normal levels of testosterone. And I test a lot

1. Jolanta Wasilewska, Maciej Kaczmarski, and Tadeusz Wasilewski, "Immunological and Non-Immunological Approaches to Dietetic Interventions in Infertility Treatment," *Sveikatos mokslai/Health Sciences* 21, no. 3 (2011): 40–44.

2. Päivi A. Pynnönen et al., "Gluten-Free Diet May Alleviate Depressive and Behavioural Symptoms in Adolescents with Coeliac Disease: A Prospective Follow-Up Case-Series Study," *BMC Psychiatry* 5, no. 1 (2005): 14.

3. Ram Reifen et al., "Serum Prolactin in Coeliac Disease: A Marker for Disease Activity," *Archives of Disease in Childhood* 77, no. 2 (1997): 155–157.

4. Gaurav Kapur et al., "Serum Prolactin in Celiac Disease," *Journal of Tropical Pediatrics* 50, no. 1 (2004): 37–40.

of people! BPA[5,6] and phthalates[7,8,9] in plastics, parabens in makeup,[10,11] and phytoestrogens in soy have all been shown to disrupt the endocrine system.[12] This endocrine disruption

5. Mohan Manikkam et al., "Plastics Derived Endocrine Disruptors (BPA, DEHP and DBP) Induce Epigenetic Transgenerational Inheritance of Obesity, Reproductive Disease and Sperm Epimutations," *PLOS One* 8, no. 1 (2013): e55387.

6. Beverly S. Rubin, "Bisphenol A: An Endocrine Disruptor with Widespread Exposure and Multiple Effects," *Journal of Steroid Biochemistry and Molecular Biology* 127, no. 1 (2011): 27–34.

7. Shanna H. Swan et al., "Decrease in Anogenital Distance among Male Infants with Prenatal Phthalate Exposure," *Environmental Health Perspectives* (2005): 1056–1061.

8. Shanna H. Swan, "Environmental Phthalate Exposure in Relation to Reproductive Outcomes and Other Health Endpoints in Humans," *Environmental Research* 108, no. 2 (2008): 177–184.

9. S. H. Swan et al., "First Trimester Phthalate Exposure and Anogenital Distance in Newborns." *Human Reproduction* 30, no. 4 (2015): 963–972.

10. Julie Boberg et al., "Possible Endocrine Disrupting Effects of Parabens and Their Metabolites," *Reproductive Toxicology* 30, no. 2 (2010): 301–312.

11. Monica Giulivo et al., "Human Exposure to Endocrine Disrupting Compounds: Their Role in Reproductive Systems, Metabolic Syndrome and Breast Cancer; A Review," *Environmental Research* 151 (2016): 251–264.

12. Timo Siepmann et al., "Hypogonadism and Erectile Dysfunction Associated with Soy Product Consumption," *Nutrition* 27, no. 7 (2011): 859–862.

from environmental toxins can increase, mimic, block, or alter the normal production of hormones.

These three causes of hormone imbalance—stress, diet, and the environment—show up mainly in Western civilization.

People who live in a more natural environment tend to have better hormonal regulation. For example, I once tested the hormones of a woman who lived in a very remote location, and her hormone balance was incredibly unique. Every part of her endocrine system was working at an optimal level. Some patients, if they are very careful with what they eat and live totally healthy lives, may be able to keep their hormones on point without intervention.

That said, I'm not going to tell you that the only way to get better is to move off the grid, eat an all-organic raw diet, and live in Shangri-La. Or to stop using plastic wrap or stop working. The goal here is to create fewer obstacles to overcome—not more of them.

Even with stressful environments, diets, and lives, we can still achieve hormone balance. We'll cover how all of this can be managed better in later chapters—so that you can not only live but thrive.

The Psychology of Hormones

Modern society is the synthesis of poor diet, stress, and compromised environment. It molds the deepest parts of ourselves—our hormones.

In today's society, women are working more[13]—often for less money than their male counterparts—and are still expected to maintain an unequal burden of household responsibilities. This results in a lot of stress, which causes that shift in how hormones respond in the body.

Modern society then goes on to add further insult to injury by adding in the stigma of women and hormones.

Your emotions are blamed on your hormones, which invalidates your authentic feelings. You are conditioned to believe you can control your emotions through sheer force of will. You're painted as "hysterical" if you can't, and an ice queen if you can. So many women come into my office and apologize about the symptoms they are experiencing *because* of the stress of trying to manage it all, as though it were a personal choice they made.

As a woman, you are told by TV shows and popular media that this is normal.

Every day, I see women who are embarrassed to talk about themselves. I can't count how many times I've heard a

---

13. Danielle Kurtzleben, "Charts: How American Men and Women Spend Their Time," *U.S. News & World Report*, June 24, 2013, 5:06 p.m. EDT.

woman start our consultation by saying, "I'm sorry, but I'm having these weird symptoms." These women apologize to me because they are not feeling well!

When I ask a female patient if she is under stress, she will invariably say, "No, of course not." But then as I question her further, her answers reveal that of course she is—often, she has been living under extreme stress for a long time. And she thinks that is just the way she is supposed to live.

I'm here to tell you that it is not.

It is not normal. You don't have to live like this. And you are not crazy.

You know your body. And you know when something feels wrong. You're not lying, you're not making anything up, and you're not complaining when you go to your doctor because something is off. These are real biological issues you are experiencing. They are based on scientific fact. They can be treated with basic medicine.

Once you own that truth, you can move forward and reclaim a productive, empowered, and healthy life.

Overcoming Trauma

One of the worst effects of modern society is inflicting shame on women who have had a traumatic experience.

And statistics show that most women have experienced trauma at some point in their lives.

Sixty percent of women have had an inappropriate sexual encounter by the time they graduate high school. One out of every six women will be a victim of attempted or complete rape in her lifetime.[14] One in five female high school students reports being physically and/or sexually abused by her partner.[15]

And those are just the cases that are reported.

Only 36 percent of rapes and 34 percent of attempted rapes are ever reported. That number is even lower for sexual assault—just 26 percent.[16]

These women and girls experience post-traumatic stress disorder (PTSD), a phenomenon that occurs when something happens to you that your body knows isn't right. Your brain doesn't have the capacity to process it, perhaps because you're too young, the event was too recent, or too many things happened at once. Your brain absorbs it without

14. National Institute of Justice and Centers for Disease Control and Prevention, Prevalence, Incidence and Consequences of Violence Against Women survey (1998).

15. J. G. Silverman et al., "Dating Violence against Adolescent Girls and Associated Substance Use, Unhealthy Weight Control, Sexual Risk Behavior, Pregnancy, and Suicidality," *Journal of the American Medical Association* 286, no. 5 (August 2001).

16. C. M. Rennison, "Rape and Sexual Assault: Reporting to Police and Medical Attention, 1992–2000," Washington, DC: U.S. Department of Justice, Bureau of Justice Statistics, August 2002, NCJ 194530.

processing it, similar to swallowing a piece of food without chewing it.

This partially processed experience sits in your head, just like a heavy lump of food in your stomach.

With PTSD, whenever you interact with someone or something linked to that experience, you have a memory of that trauma. It's not always sexual. It can be caused by verbal abuse, emotional abuse, the way you were raised, even abuse at work.

That stress becomes a part of you. It manifests in your body—showing up in the form of trust issues, panic attacks, problems with libido, or abnormal weight gain. Not only do you have the injury of your trauma, but society heaps further shame upon you by admonishing you for not controlling your body. You've had that control taken away from you.

But when you start to balance your hormones again, you take back that control. You can't avoid your stressors or your trauma anymore. And you don't want to avoid it—you want to deal with it. You want to come to terms with it. You get the help you need to process it.

And that is the most empowering step of all.

Take Back Control

When you take control of your health, you take control of your life. But you can't take control until you know what to look for.

In the upcoming chapters, we are going to look at the most common hormones in your body, the ways in which these hormones may become out of balance, and treatment for hormone imbalance.

Know your body, know your mind. When we talk about hormones, it's incredibly important to understand the basics of body and brain chemistry. You need to understand the impact the body has on the mind. That knowledge empowers you to break out of feeling guilty about your symptoms, and to reject the belief that feeling bad is normal. You can then start to make positive changes.

Estrogen and progesterone. Biologically, estrogen and progesterone comprise the two halves of what it means to be a woman. But estrogen is widely misunderstood, while progesterone is chronically deficient. For many women, achieving the correct balance between these two hormones alone can be life changing.

Thyroid. Your thyroid is the thermostat of your metabolism. Thyroid plays a role in weight, cognitive function, memory, and mental acuity. When it's turned up, the higher metabolism helps your digestion, immune system, and cardiovascular system. When it's off, things don't run smoothly. A balanced thyroid plays a key role in helping to balance your hormones.

Testosterone. Far from being just for men, testosterone supports your libido, confidence, assertiveness, aggressiveness, risk taking, and boundary setting. Without healthy testosterone levels, you will have a much harder time going after the life you want to build. This is why testosterone is such a crucial part of hormone balance.

Neurotransmitters. Neurotransmitters are the messages around your brain associated with your moods, emotional state, and mental wellness. Hormone balance directly affects your neurotransmitters. When this relationship is healthy, you can feel the difference.

Treatments. Treatment for hormone balance is not "one size fits all." It involves testing to figure out where the imbalance is so you can correct it. It also involves learning how to communicate with your doctor to get the best health care possible. You need to become your own advocate, because you know your body better than anyone does.

Hormone imbalance is a dynamic interplay within your body, but it's not hard to correct. You don't have to put your life on hold to address it. I treat women every day who continue to work and move forward in this world, productive and empowered and healthy.

You can be one of these women as well.

You can keep living your life *and* do away with mood swings and other symptoms of hormone imbalance at the same time. You just need to know how to monitor these aspects of your health in order to manage them. When you do, you can give yourself the freedom to live your life the way you want and to make it the best it can be.

The first step is to go back to the basics. In the next chapter, we will run through a crash course about your body and your mind and how the two influence each other.

Chapter 2

Know Your Body, Know Your Mind

Julie's Story

I want to share with you the story of a woman named Julie.

Her hormone story begins at age thirteen, when Julie experiences her first period. Her menstrual cycle is complicated and irregular, with cramping over the first few days. Her mother assures her this is normal. But when Julie begins missing a day of school every month, her parents take her to see the family doctor.

"These symptoms are normal for a girl your age," he tells her, and he prescribes oral contraceptive pills for the cramps. Julie's parents are confused. She is not sexually active, so why would the doctor prescribe a contraceptive for her period? They ultimately assume that their doctor would warn them of any significant side effects, and they fill the prescription.

By college, Julie no longer has difficult periods, but she feels as if she has to be very strict with her diet to prevent weight gain. When Julie brings this up at the campus clinic, the nurse assures her that the weight gain has nothing to do with the birth control pills. "Just exercise more and eat less," advises the nurse. Also during this time, Julie realizes that she does not have a healthy libido. She finds herself less and less interested in intimacy.

Julie graduates, begins her career, and at twenty-six meets a guy and falls in love. They get married. Two years later, she stops her birth control. By age twenty-nine, she conceives her first child.

Julie experiences postpartum depression. She feels robbed of the elation she expected to feel after the birth of her child: she had pictured an idyllic time bonding with and loving her newborn. When she reports this to her obstetrician, he assures her that this is normal for a woman who just gave birth, and he prescribes Zoloft for six months.

Over the next four years, Julie stays off birth control and conceives two more children. After each childbirth, she experiences the same depression and is prescribed Zoloft. Her doctor advises her to stay on the Zoloft as a preventative. The only time she stops is when she is trying to conceive and when she is pregnant.

Being a stay-at-home mother of three is stressful. Julie has occasionally had anxiety in her life, mostly with her periods, but now she begins to feel that anxiety in waves. She can't ignore it, so she brings it up with her doctor. He prescribes Xanax.

By thirty-five, Julie stops taking Zoloft, gets back on birth control, and goes back to work. She works harder than ever before. Every morning, Julie wakes up early to exercise and then gets the kids up and ready for school and sees them out the door. She puts in a full day at the office and then shuttles the kids to after-school activities before coming home to supervise homework while making dinner. After dinner, she cleans the kitchen, puts the kids to bed, and folds laundry while watching TV. Then she falls into bed and gets up early to start all over again.

Julie is often tired and finds herself drinking more coffee in the morning along with energy drinks in the afternoon. She is also more irritable than before. Her husband complains that she doesn't have time for him. They fight more often, usually over nothing of consequence.

Since college, Julie has worked hard to keep her weight in the healthy range. This all changes in her forties, when she gains a significant amount of weight. Her routine of careful diet and regular exercise no longer works for her. She restricts her diet to one thousand calories per day and trains for and completes several local 5K and 10K races. But Julie still can't keep her weight under control.

By her mid-forties, Julie experiences insomnia, low libido, fatigue, and depression. Her periods become more irregular, and now they're painful. Instead of three to four days, they now last seven to ten days and are heavier than ever. She feels tired and drained.

Her physician listens to the list of symptoms, runs a battery of tests, and tells her she is "fine." He says it is normal for her period to be irregular at this point in her life. He changes her birth control, prescribes Ambien for sleep, recommends going back on Zoloft, and renews her prescription for Xanax. "Don't forget that you need to eat less and exercise more," he reminds her. He also implies that if she lost weight, her libido would return.

Julie wants to ask, "What happened to my life? What happened to my body? What happened to my zest, my happiness? Why do I need all these medications—and then when I take them, I *still* feel crazy?"

Could there have been another way? she wonders.

The Owner's Manual

Julie is an amalgam of many patients I have seen. Her story is a universal and depressing one. As you read through the rest of this book, see if you recognize Julie—or yourself. Her plight occurs because, too often, doctors focus only on a patient's symptoms. They don't apply themselves to the question of *why* she has those symptoms to begin with.

This is where we step in.

We are going to jump off this swing. And it begins by understanding what is happening in your body and mind, and taking charge of both.

You may be asking yourself, "Why is this so important? I've lived in this body all my life. Don't I know everything I really need to know about it by now?"

Think of the information in this chapter as the owner's manual to your body.

When you learn how to drive, you are taught the basics of a car and how it works. You need to know where the engine is, that it has brakes, and how the steering wheel controls the four tires. After that, you learn about which gasoline to put in it and why. You learn about oil and how it keeps the engine running. You may even choose to discover more about the finer systems that work within your vehicle.

And just as you need this information before you get behind the wheel, you also need to know the basics of your body and its functions.

This information orients you within the systems of your body. With that understanding, you also take control of your mind and understand what to do when one of those systems misfires.

You take your car to a mechanic for tune-ups. Similarly, you see your doctor to keep everything running smoothly in your body. Once you understand your body's different parts and how they work together, you can make educated decisions about your health. You can have effective conversations with your doctor to help you get everything back in balance.

You are empowered to take control of your body, your mind, and your life.

In this chapter, we will cover the physical parts of your body, including your brain, and how they work. We'll also break down eleven of the hormones and neurotransmitters that affect your body and mind the most.

Body Parts

The physical parts of your body may seem pretty basic—hey, we all have them, right?—but most of us don't understand exactly how those parts work. Knowing your body, as a woman, begins with understanding the four main parts of your endocrine system: your ovaries, adrenal glands, thyroid, and brain.

Ovaries and Menstrual Cycle

When it comes to ovaries, the main biological process to understand is the menstrual cycle. A good metaphor for the female menstrual cycle is the four seasons of the year.

Think of the very beginning of your cycle (the days right after the end of your period) as winter. All your hormones are quiet, and everything operates at a low level. When your brain senses that quiet, it surges with a hormone from the anterior pituitary called follicle-stimulating hormone, or FSH. FSH jumps down to your ovaries and stimulates them to wake up.

This begins the springtime. When FSH rises and stimulates the ovaries, it specifically stimulates follicles in the ovaries that release estrogen. For the next two weeks, estrogen rises and travels to all the parts of your body that define you as a woman, with the goal of preparing the body to conceive: the glandular tissue in your breasts, healthy mucosa in your cervix and vaginal tissue, adipose cells around your hips and breasts, and finally back to the ovaries themselves. That growth and stimulation increases blood flow to these areas and builds up the tissue that lines your uterus, getting it ready to implant an egg.

Once your estrogen hits its apex, the brain flips a switch and stops the FSH. Here we enter summer.

At this point in the cycle, both FSH and estrogen drop immediately. As FSH drops, the body releases luteinizing hormone, or LH. LH then signals the ovaries to release an egg. Once the egg is released, support follicles are transformed into corpora lutea, the role of which is to secrete progesterone.

Progesterone rises up to balance your estrogen. It goes back to the same tissue estrogen stimulated and tempers its growth to keep the tissue healthy and prevent excessive stimulation. During this time of autumn, progesterone slows the growth and stimulation of the ovaries, fat cells, and lining of your uterus. This lasts for an equal amount of time as spring, when your estrogen rises, and it prevents that growth from causing damage to your body.

If a fertilized egg doesn't implant in the lining of the uterus, progesterone and LH drop off. This signals the body to begin menstruation, and then everything goes quiet again—back to winter.

As a woman ages, ovulation begins to slow down and becomes less consistent, usually in the mid- to late thirties. In fact, it doesn't always occur with each cycle. If ovulation is weak, a woman generates less progesterone. If she doesn't ovulate at all, her progesterone will be minimal at best, and estrogen will be dominant. This can be due to stress, poor diet, or environmental factors. This deficiency of progesterone can affect serotonin, melatonin, and GABA—which we will cover later in this chapter.

Adrenal Glands

Your adrenal glands, which sit atop each kidney, contribute to the daily rhythm of your life.

One of the tasks of your adrenal glands is to produce the hormone cortisol. Your body has an internal clock that wakes you up in the morning with a surge of cortisol. As the day progresses, cortisol naturally starts to decline. Once it hits its lowest point, you fall asleep again.

Your body secretes more cortisol, a natural anti-inflammatory, when it is under stress. Your body can handle light stimulation of cortisol, but chronic stimulation of this hormone over time causes more health problems.

Some stress is good. If you go to the gym and kick butt, that's good stress. But if you feel stressed day in and day out, and every day is a grind, you can hit a point where your level of cortisol is chronically elevated. Chronic elevations of cortisol can inhibit ovulation. Cortisol is also neuro-toxic, so it damages brain tissue over time. This cognitive decline means you can't think as clearly. Chronic cortisol elevation triggers long-term weight gain by causing insulin resistance.

If this hypercortisol period goes on for a long time, the adrenal glands experience fatigue and drop off the produc-tion of cortisol. This leads to a hypocortisol stage, where you're just exhausted all the time.

Thyroid

The thyroid is basically the dimmer switch of your metabolism.

A small, butterfly-shaped gland located in your neck, your thyroid sits right in front of your esophagus. Further up, in the pituitary gland in your brain, lives a thermostat that measures how much thyroid hormone you have at any one time and adjusts accordingly.

Your pituitary gland maintains hormone balance for all of the parts of the endocrine system. You can think of this as the thermostat for the heater in your house. If the ther-mostat reads that the heat is too low, the heater turns on. If the pituitary gland thinks you're low on thyroid hormone, it sends a signal to the thyroid gland.

The signal to your thyroid is thyroid stimulating hormone, or TSH.

Though it seems counterintuitive, the higher your TSH, the lower your active thyroid hormone level: when your thyroid hormone level drops, your TSH increases as a signal to your thyroid. Once your thyroid receives that signal, it creates thyroxine, or T4. This precursor hormone is not biologically active at all. Once it reaches the liver and muscles, T4 is converted into triiodothyronine, or T3, which is the active hormone that binds to the surface of your cells and fires up your metabolism.

As we age, the pituitary sends less and less TSH to the thyroid. Our bodies basically try to slow down our metabolism, kind of like putting us in hibernation. This decline of the thyroid is a slow process, which leads to decreased metabolism and cognition. We will discuss this further in chapter 4.

Brain

Your brain takes food in the form of protein and coverts it into neurotransmitters. Neurotransmitters are the messages that neurons send to each other, affecting your mood.

If you have too many neurotransmitters firing at once, you are unable to focus your attention and may experience symptoms similar to ADHD, or attention deficit/hyperactivity disorder. Most people, however, experience a deficiency issue with their neurotransmitters, which causes the enzyme pathway to slow down. When this happens, you can't think clearly.

Sometimes the biochemical pathways in the brain are irregular. And in some of us, they are so irregular that we can't compensate when placed in a stressful situation. As we age, the system breaks down further, leading to more neurotransmitter deficiencies.

Hormones directly influence neurotransmitters. Hormone fluctuations can explain symptoms of anxiety, depression, and insomnia. While hormone imbalance is a common cause of neurotransmitter irregularities, sometimes the brain chemistry itself is off. Again, we will discuss this further in our discussion of neurotransmitters in chapter 6.

Know Your Hormones (and Neurotransmitters)

Now that you are more familiar with the physical parts of your body, you're ready to get to know your hormones and neurotransmitters themselves a little better. You can think of this list as an introduction to—or dictionary of terms for—eleven of the most important chemical messengers in your body. We'll be covering these in more depth in later chapters.

Estrogen. There are three different types of estrogen: estradiol, estrone, and estriol. These are beautiful hormones and are responsible for the feminine part of your identity. We will discuss each of them further in chapter 3.

Progesterone. Progesterone is the most important hormone I talk about with my patients. It balances estrogen's growth. It also plays an intimate role in your brain chemistry. Progesterone is so important because it is the most chronically deficient hormone due to the modern lifestyle. We will also examine this hormone more in the next chapter.

Testosterone. Women are supposed to have testosterone, just as men are supposed to have estrogen. It is a misunderstood, forgotten hormone for women, but it is very important to your biochemistry. Testosterone is produced in the adrenal glands and ovaries. We will discuss its effect on your body in greater detail in chapter 5.

Cortisol. Cortisol, a steroid, is the most fundamental hormone the body makes. It is the body's natural anti-inflammatory agent. As we discussed earlier, cortisol is related to stress. It also increases blood sugar and modulates the immune system. Cortisol affects the metabolism of fats, carbohydrates, and protein. It also affects bone density.

Thyroid stimulating hormone (TSH). Thyroid stimulating hormone is generated in the brain and works as the messenger between the pituitary and thyroid glands. TSH tells the thyroid to produce thyroxine.

Triiodothyronine (T3). T3 is like a metabolic explosion in your body. It is super active, strong, and effective. T3 is the hormone that touches tissue and makes things happen in your metabolism.

Thyroxine (T4). If T3 is the explosion, T4 is a hand grenade before you pull the pin. It is the step just before you make T3 active. Without being active, T4 is completely inert.

Serotonin. Serotonin is a mood balancer and the most common neurotransmitter in your digestive system. Serotonin creates the "gut feeling" that people often describe.

Serotonin starts off as an amino acid, called tryptophan, in the food you eat. When tryptophan crosses the blood-brain barrier, it turns into 5-hydroxytryptophan. This pathway is influenced by progesterone. Progesterone enhances the production of serotonin. Serotonin deficiency can be caused by an issue with an enzyme that interferes with the conversion process.

People think of serotonin primarily as the hormone associated with depression, but low serotonin can cause other problems as well. Serotonin deficiency is the most common cause of migraines and a common cause of sugar cravings. Low serotonin levels can also cause digestive problems during your period.

Melatonin. Serotonin eventually turns into melatonin. Without progesterone, that conversion is impaired. And if you have low serotonin, you will develop low melatonin. Melatonin is the neurotransmitter that strongly helps regulate the pineal gland, which puts you into a circadian rhythm of sleep. Low melatonin levels can cause insomnia.

GABA. Glutamine in your diet turns into glutamic acid, which then turns into gamma-aminobutyric acid, or GABA. GABA is a neurotransmitter that inhibits the transmission of nerve impulses in the central nervous system. Basically, it is your natural antianxiety agent.

Anxiety is caused by having too many signals firing in your brain all at once. GABA is like a shock absorber. It throttles back the signals in your brain to calm down the flood of information.

Sex hormone binding globulin. Sex hormone binding globulin is a protein made by your liver. It is your body's way of protecting itself by preventing you from having too much of an active hormone in your body at any given time. However, balance is important with sex hormone binding globulin. If you have too much, it gobbles up all the active testosterone in your body. And if it's too low, you can have too much active testosterone.

Time for a Tune-Up

We've covered mind-body basics in this chapter. But the truth is, there is always more to learn about your body and your mind.

Take Julie's story. Her life might have been very different if she had understood the interactions among her hormones, her brain, and the rest of her body.

For example, when Julie was young, she was not ovulating. This caused heavy bleeding due to excessive estrogen stimulation without the balancing effect of progesterone. Her testosterone was diminished due to oral birth control, which spiked the amount of sex hormone binding globulin she had. Julie gained weight in college, and her libido diminished as she aged.

During pregnancy, Julie had super high progesterone. When she gave birth, it went to zero. That drop caused her postpartum depression. Her progesterone deficiency led to a serotonin deficiency. Julie's depression wasn't caused by low Zoloft levels!

Chronic stress through her thirties and into her forties, due to an unhealthy work-home life balance, caused cortisol weight gain, leaving her unable to lose weight with diet alone. Her dry skin, cold hands, and slow weight gain were all influenced by low thyroid. Continued low progesterone threw off her GABA, causing anxiety.

At each encounter, instead of being informed by her doctor, Julie was given a pill or told to ignore her symptoms. But these weren't personal flaws. Julie's experience wasn't something she made up in her mind. At no point did her physician address the physiological evidence in front of him that proved something was wrong.

That's just not right.

Knowing your body and knowing your mind means going beyond the belief that "this is just the way things are." The new story goes, "This is my body, and this is what it does to my mind and my mood. What do I need to do to correct this biological problem?"

And that's what we're going to look at next.

You are now more familiar with your body and your mind. But what exactly do you do if one or both feels off? In the upcoming chapters, we are going to take a look at specific hormones and other causes of imbalance, along with the symptoms of each. It all starts in the next chapter with the yin and yang of hormones: estrogen and progesterone.

Chapter 3

Estrogen and Progesterone

Birth and Destruction

The two most famous goddesses in the Greek and Roman pantheons are Venus and Athena.

The goddess of love, who is called Venus or Aphrodite, is best known for her beauty, sexuality, and fertility. She has been painted by everyone from Sandro Botticelli to Henri Pierre Picou. These artistic impressions tend to have a few things in common. We most often see Venus with long, flowing hair and soft curves. She usually isn't wearing many clothes, and she seems to enjoy lounging on oversized clamshells.

And then we have Athena.

Athena is the goddess of wisdom and war. Unlike Venus, Athena doesn't just wear clothes; she decks herself out in full-body armor and carries a spear. The paintings we see of Athena are a lot less about lounging and a lot more about standing tall on a mountaintop, looking upon the conquered world at her feet.

Venus and Athena are polar opposites. But in mythology, each commands equal respect.

Because you are a woman, these two forces—love and wisdom, birth and destruction—are at work in your body as we speak. Only these days, instead of referring to them as Venus and Athena, we have more scientific names for them: estrogen and progesterone.

We Go Together

Why are estrogen and progesterone so important? And why is it important to talk about these two hormones at the same time, rather than independently?

In the hormone world, estrogen and progesterone are the two halves that define what it means to be a woman. They work together as a unit. Estrogen and progesterone are more closely associated with feminine health than any other hormones in the body.

So what are they, exactly?

Estrogen is the beautiful, feminizing, fertile part of you—your "Venus" hormone. Progesterone, meanwhile, is the part of you associated with better brain chemistry, mood, energy, and sense of self—your "Athena" hormone.

While estrogen is all about growth, progesterone can be seen as its counterbalance to modulate estrogen's stimulation in your body. When these levels are not balanced, a lot can go wrong. Your body can become flooded with excesses—autoimmune responses, hyperstimulation of the uterus and breast—which can lead to tissue overgrowth, high blood sugar, insulin resistance, vaginal infections, and obesity.

When estrogen and progesterone are in balance, however, your body can keep these systems in check, allowing your health to flourish. The body's ability to control and modulate growth represents the height of evolution.

But how exactly do estrogen and progesterone work in your body? Let's take a closer look at each.

The Estrogen Triad

Estrogen comes in three forms. In order of strength, they are estradiol, estrone, and estriol.

Estradiol is the most feminizing estrogen. It stimulates breast and ovarian tissue as well as the lining of your uterus. It also stimulates adipose cells, which give you curves and help define the feminine form. Estradiol helps make HDL cholesterol, which protects you against atherosclerosis and heart attacks, builds bone density, and strengthens the attachments of tendons. It is also essential for your vaginal ecology.

Estrone is a downstream metabolite of estradiol. Your ovaries make estradiol, which circulates in the body. Once estradiol finishes its job of promoting growth, it is converted to estrone by the body's fat cells. Estrone then works its way into your liver, which detoxifies the estrone and eliminates it. Estrone is not a feminizing estrogen. On the contrary, when it is elevated, it stimulates thrombin, which causes deep vein thrombosis and clots. Estrone is also linked to breast pain, breast cancer, nausea, hypertension, and leg cramps.

Estriol, a weak hormone, gets elevated during pregnancy. Some doctors believe it can help with menopausal symptoms, though we would have to use so much of it that its use is not reasonable. However, a 2002 study from UCLA found that estriol can put multiple sclerosis into remission.[17]

Often, doctors request only total estrogen on lab work. However, this lab will provide only one piece of the puzzle. To understand the full picture of your estrogen imbalance, you will want to ask for a test to look at the breakdown of all three estrogens. Understanding the three types is key to having a productive discussion about estrogen balance with your doctor.

Real versus Fake Progesterone

Meanwhile, as we've already touched on, progesterone serves to counterbalance estrogen. Your ovaries release progesterone in the middle of your cycle. When progesterone crosses

---

17. Nancy L. Sicotte et al., "Treatment of Multiple Sclerosis with the Pregnancy Hormone Estriol," *Annals of Neurology* 52, no. 4 (2002): 421–428.

the blood-brain barrier, it turns into 5-allo-pregnenolone, which binds to the GABA receptors in your brain. GABA is your natural antianxiety agent; therefore, progesterone acts like a shock absorber, dampening any discordance and making things calmer. Without progesterone stimulating your GABA receptors, your brain moves toward anxiety, whether you want it to or not.

Progesterone also plays a role in the production of monoamines such as serotonin and melatonin. Without progesterone, your ability to generate serotonin and melatonin is reduced.

Oral contraceptives are made of powerful synthetic hormones. These synthetic hormones, at high doses, inhibit the production of progesterone and provide synthetic progesterone as a substitute. Synthetic progesterone is also given as hormone replacement therapy in postmenopausal women.

But synthetic progesterone can be dangerous.

The molecular structure of synthetic progesterone, called medroxyprogesterone acetate, or MPA, is different from that of natural progesterone. It is similar, but the difference is significant. Both medroxyprogesterone acetate and natural progesterone are made up of four rings. The difference comes with the addition of an acetyl group to make medroxyprogesterone acetate. This added group changes the dynamic of the compound.

Medroxyprogesterone acetate's strange structure binds well to the lining of the uterus, but not to the breasts or the brain. Synthetic progesterone will not calm the mind. It will not bind to the GABA receptor. And it will not help make serotonin or melatonin. In fact, medroxyprogesterone acetate actually blocks natural progesterone from binding to the GABA receptor, and it inhibits progesterone from promoting serotonin and melatonin.[18]

Think of it as Dr. Jekyll and Mr. Hyde: one helps keep you sane, while the other makes you feel crazy.

Striking the right balance between estrogen and progesterone is critical. They are responsible for bringing balance to your body. Keeping their levels equalized allows you to live a fulfilling life in which you can be your happiest self.

Before we can balance progesterone and estrogen, however, we first need to demystify progesterone and remove some of the stigma surrounding estrogen.

Demystifying Progesterone

A low level of progesterone, your Athena hormone, is the most common hormone deficiency in women, hands down.

Progesterone is essential for conception. The Latin term for progesterone means "pro-gestation," or "hold the

---

18. T. Rabe, L. Kiesel, and B. Runnebaum, *Antiprogestins*, in Actions of Progesterone on the Brain, ed. D. Ganten and D. Pfaff, Current Topics in Neuroendocrinology, vol. 5. (Berlin: Springer-Verlag, 1985).

pregnancy." As you age, your body alters your progesterone levels. This most commonly occurs in your early thirties.

While aging leads to natural decreases in progesterone, it's not the only reason you may be experiencing low progesterone levels.

As I mentioned in chapter 1, the epidemic of stress in modern culture is a significant cause of progesterone deficiency. When you're under stress, your body doesn't generate progesterone, and it doesn't ovulate because it doesn't want you to conceive during stress. The second cause of progesterone deficiency is diet, and the third is environment and toxins.

Progesterone deficiency causes most of the symptoms that are unique to women.

An unhealthy estrogen-progesterone ratio can cause you to store body fat disproportionately, creating a skewed waist-hip ratio. It can be easier to gain weight and more difficult to lose it. You may also feel like your breasts are overly swollen during menses.

Without progesterone, estrogen hyperstimulates breast tissue to grow, causing breast pain. Studies show that after sixty months of cyclic breast pain, risk factors for breast cancer go through the roof.[19] Low progesterone, associated

---

19. G. Plu-Bureau et al., "Cyclical Mastalgia as a Marker of Breast Cancer Susceptibility: Results of a Case-Control Study among French Women," *British Journal of Cancer* 65, no. 6 (June 1992): 945–949.

with polycystic ovarian syndrome (PCOS), increases the risk factors for breast cancer, ovarian cancer, and uterine cancer.[20,21,22,23,24,25,26,27]

Natural progesterone is the most powerful anticancer agent for reproductive cancers. Progesterone induces

20. Matthew J. Carlson, "Catch It before It Kills: Progesterone, Obesity, and the Prevention of Endometrial Cancer," *Discovery Medicine* 14, no.76 (2012): 215.

21. Harvey A. Risch, "Hormonal Etiology of Epithelial Ovarian Cancer, with a Hypothesis Concerning the Role of Androgens and Progesterone," *Journal of the National Cancer Institute* 90, no. 23 (1998): 1774–1786.

22. J. Foidart et al., "Estradiol and Progesterone Regulate the Proliferation of Human Breast Epithelial Cells," *Fertility and Sterility* 69, no. 5 (1998): 963–969.

23. H. Franke and I. Vermes, "Differential Effects of Progestogens on Breast Cancer Cell Lines," *Maturitas* 46 (2003): 55–58.

24. G. Colditz, "Estrogen, Estrogen Plus Progestin Therapy, and Risk of Breast Cancer," *Clinical Cancer Research* 11 (2005): 909–917.

25. A. Fournier, F. Berrino, and F. Clavel-Chapelon, "Unequal Risks for Breast Cancer Associated with Different Hormone Replacement Therapies: Results from the E3N Cohort Study," Abstract, *Breast Cancer Research and Treatment* 107, no. 1 (2008) 103–111.

26. B. De Lignières et al., "Combined Hormone Replacement Therapy and Risk of Breast Cancer in a French Cohort Study of 3175 Women," Abstract, *Climacteric* 5 (2002): 332–340.

27. Plu-Bureau et al., "Cyclical Mastalgia," 945–949.

apoptosis, or cell death, in breast, ovarian, endometrial, and uterine cancer cells.[28,29,30,31]

Just as progesterone plays a role in your physical identity, it can affect your mental identity as well. This goes back to the GABA receptors in your brain, which progesterone modulates. When this relationship is out of whack, you're going to have anxiety.

Statistically, women experience more anxiety and depression than men do.[32] These are both symptoms of progesterone deficiency. In an average year, during which time I see thousands of people, I normally have only one or two cases

28. Hisham et al., "Progesterone Receptor Modulates ER [agr] Action in Breast Cancer," *Nature* 523, no. 7560 (2015): 313–317.

29. Valerie C. L. Lin et al., "Effect of Progesterone on the Invasive Properties and Tumor Growth of Progesterone Receptor-Transfected Breast Cancer Cells MDA-MB-231," *Clinical Cancer Research* 7, no. 9 (2001): 2880–2886.

30. Stanley G. Korenman, "The Endocrinology of Breast Cancer," *Cancer* 46, no. S4 (1980): 874–878.

31. Bent Formby and T. S. Wiley, "Progesterone Inhibits Growth and Induces Apoptosis in Breast Cancer Cells: Inverse Effects on Bcl-2 and p53," *Annals of Clinical and Laboratory Science* 28, no. 6 (1998): 360–369.

32. C. P. McLean et al., "Gender Differences in Anxiety Disorders: Prevalence, Course of Illness, Comorbidity and Burden of Illness," *Journal of Psychiatric Research* 45, no. 8 (2011):1027–1035. doi:10.1016/j.jpsychires.2011.03.006.

in which anxiety and depression aren't related to a progesterone deficiency.

Once you bring progesterone back to a healthy level in your body, your brain is able to do what it's naturally meant to do again.

Destigmatizing Estrogen

The whole world operates with a very dualistic mindset. Something is either good or it's bad, with no middle ground. Estrogen has been painted with this black-and-white brush.

Women's bodies, however, are not binary.

Estrogen often gets vilified due to oversimplification, especially when it comes to cancer. Too much estrogen causes problems like cancer, right? And we remove the estrogen when there's a problem, right? Therefore, estrogen must be the problem.

Except it's not always that simple.

Estrogen needs to be metabolized to be effective. It is your liver's job to reduce estrogen levels by the end of your cycle. But many people consume foods either containing added estrogens or contaminated with plastics that have estrogen actions. Other people eat a diet low in fiber, but fiber is a necessary part of estrogen elimination. Some people don't metabolize estrogens very well, so they're stuck with elevated levels of the less-healthy version of estrogen: estrone.

Allow me to be a little controversial: estrogen does not cause cancer.[33,34] But when you have too little progesterone, you can have a higher risk for developing cancer.[35] By definition, cancer is an overgrowth, and progesterone's job in the body is to prevent overgrowth. If someone already has a type of cancer that is estrogen-receptor active, estrogen will make the cancer worse. But again, it is not the presence of estrogen that causes the problem. It's the lack of progesterone.

Despite these facts, estrogen is demonized, misunderstood, and made to be something that it's not.

Estrogen is the scapegoat. Just like the last kid to leave the playroom gets blamed for the mess—even if lots of other kids helped make it—estrogen is blamed for issues like

33. J.-M. Foidart et al., "Estradiol and Progesterone Regulate the Proliferation of Human Breast Epithelial Cells," *Fertility and Sterility* 69, no. 5 (May 1998): 963–969. University of Liege, Belgium (n = 40 postmenopausal women => biopsies).

34. L. J. Hofseth, "Hormone Replacement Therapy with Estrogen or Estrogen Plus Medroxyprogesterone Acetate Is Associated with Increased Epithelial Proliferation in the Normal Postmenopausal Breast," *Journal of Clinical Endocrinology and Metabolism* 84, no. 12 (December 1999): 4559–4565. Department of Physiology, Michigan State University, East Lansing, MI 48824, US (n = 86 postmenopausal women).

35. Stanley G. Korenman, "Oestrogen Window Hypothesis of the Aetiology of Breast Cancer," *Lancet* 315, no. 8170 (1980): 700–701.

cancer, just for being present. Meanwhile, progesterone is ignored.

But when looking at hormone imbalance, it is always important to remember that estrogen and progesterone go hand in hand.

The Deficiency Duo

When estrogen and progesterone levels are off, we must examine the role of both hormones.

In regard to estrogen and progesterone imbalance in women, I generally see two main pathologies: progesterone deficiency with normal estradiol, or progesterone deficiency with raised estradiol. And the symptoms fall anywhere along a continuum.

With too little progesterone and normal estradiol, you may have occasional missed periods. Your estrogen levels have not become elevated enough for breast pain with your cycle, ovarian cysts, or heavy, painful periods. You most likely experience mental and emotional symptoms, such as irritability and insomnia.

With low progesterone and high estradiol, you probably don't ovulate often. Estrogen builds up in your body, causing ovarian symptoms such as PCOS, uterine symptoms such as painful periods, and breast pathology including pain and cysts. You are more likely to experience anxiety and depression.

Women with too much estradiol are uniquely feminine. Their symptoms get worse with their periods, pointing to excessive stimulation of their reproductive tissues. Their treatment requires much more aggressive doses of progesterone than what is needed by women with normal or low estrogen levels. They have so much estrogen naturally occurring that they need more help maintaining balance.

Once you rebalance your hormone levels, your life will regain its balance as well.

Venus and Athena

Venus and Athena, or estrogen and progesterone, are incredible in their own ways. But the key is finding the right balance between these two halves.

As beautiful as each may be on its own, estrogen and progesterone are strongest when they are working together. At your healthiest, you are more than just one or the other. You are Athena and Venus, estrogen and progesterone, love and wisdom, mind and body, both soft and strong.

When these powerful forces, which are often seen as a pendulum or a swing, are correctly balanced, you are unstoppable.

Now you know about the two dominant female hormones in your body. But what happens if these two hormones are in balance and you still feel off? It's time to take a look at your thyroid, which we'll discuss in the next chapter.

Chapter 4

Thyroid

Up and Down

Jessica had a high-stress political job working for the state of Arizona. When she came to see me in 2011, she had hypothyroid issues, weight gain, fatigue, depression, anxiety, and joint and muscle pain.

I ran a comprehensive thyroid panel and saw that Jessica had autoimmunity: her body made antibodies that were attacking her own thyroid. Jessica's autoimmune levels, specifically thyroid peroxidase antibodies, blew my mind. The normal level is below 30. Jessica's went all the way up to 1,126.

Even after we normalized her other hormone levels and adjusted her diet, we couldn't get Jessica's immune system to cooperate. So I started diving further into what was happening with her.

I learned that Jessica's work environment had become so stressful that it bordered on abusive. The severe emotional stress caused her adrenal glands to produce cortisol at extremely high levels. I referred Jessica to an endocrinologist for a second opinion, with no success. Even though it was upsetting to me to recommend this, I had to counsel her to leave her job. I was worried about the impact this toxic environment was having on her mental and physical health.

Jessica didn't feel that quitting was possible, especially after having fought so hard to rise to her position. For a long time, she regimented her life as much as she could, trying to reduce the stress. It helped a little, but her health problems never went away.

Then one day in May 2016, Jessica came to see me again. When I looked at her chart, I thought I had someone else's labs. Her thyroid peroxidase antibody level was at 172: still high, but remarkably better. I walked into the exam room, mouth agape, and just stared at Jessica. It had been three months since I had last seen her. She was radiant. Her hair was down, and it looked fuller. She had lost weight, she looked vibrant, and somehow there were fewer lines on her face. It was as though the weight of the world—not just body weight—had been lifted from her.

And I asked her, "Jessica, what changed? How did you do it?"

She smiled serenely. "I left my job."

She had pushed herself to the point of surrender. And, in that moment, she experienced a little miracle: she was offered a job in her local town government, with similar pay and none of the stress.

The next time I tested her, Jessica's thyroid antibodies were off-the-charts unmeasurable again—but this time because they were so low. And this strong woman, who had been through so much, was the picture of perfect health.

Her story only serves to illustrate the importance of that small, butterfly-shaped gland in your throat: the thyroid.

Lights, Camera, Action

As I mentioned in chapter 2, whenever I tell someone about her thyroid, I explain it as a dimmer switch in the body.

Your thyroid turns up your metabolism, stimulating your cells to be active. Your cells are always going to run, but, like a dimmer switch, the thyroid can have them running on high or on low, similar to how we can turn a dimmer switch up or down to affect the light in a room we're sitting in. When the lights are really low, our eyes will adapt within thirty minutes to that level of brightness. When we enter a regularly lit space, the room will seem really bright.

The same is true with your thyroid. People adapt to having an underactive thyroid. Once your thyroid is optimized, it's like stepping into a bright, sunny day.

An underactive thyroid causes a pervasive feeling of sluggishness, fatigue, and low energy. You gain weight disproportionately to what you eat. You don't remember things as well as you should. And you may think it's normal, associated with aging. But really, you've gotten used to a thyroid issue that has developed gradually. The thyroid incrementally decreases its function. Everything that's supposed to move slows down, even as we keep going with our busy lives.

When the thyroid does its job, it keeps a nice metabolic tone throughout your body. Everything runs at the right level of energy. You recall facts crisply. Your immune system is responsive.[36] Your body metabolizes fats and calories correctly.[37] Your hair grows thick, your nails grow long, and your skin is healthy.

Your thyroid is directly linked to every system in your body, so its health directly affects your overall health.

In this chapter, we are going to examine the thyroid's link to other systems in your body, talk about what tests to run to check your thyroid levels, and discuss diagnosis and treatment for the thyroid.

36. K. A. El-Shaikh, "Recovery of Age-Dependent Immunological Deterioration in Old Mice by Thyroxine Treatment," *Journal of Animal Physiology and Animal Nutrition (Berl)* 90, no. 5-6 (June 2006): 244–254.

37. N. Knudsen et al., "Small Differences in Thyroid Function May Be Important for Body Mass Index and the Occurrence of Obesity in the Population," *Journal of Clinical Endocrinology and Metabolism* 90, no. 7 (July 2005): 4019–4024.

All Systems Go

When your thyroid is off, it is easy to tell, because everything in your body seems to slow down. But you don't need to have outright hypothyroidism for this gland to have a noticeable impact on your whole body. Having a suboptimally functioning thyroid can cause serious symptoms.

Let's take a deeper look at how your thyroid interacts with your cardiovascular, immunological, hepatic, neurological, and digestive systems.

Cardiovascular

The thyroid plays an important role in cardiovascular health.

When your thyroid is functioning in the suboptimal range, specifically when free T3 is below 3.2,[38] you have a higher risk factor for mortality associated with a cardiovascular event, even if you don't have preexisting heart issues. And if you do have heart problems, your thyroid at its optimal level can save your life.

Your thyroid is meant to protect your heart. If you were to have a heart attack, your thyroid gland would help remodel

---

38. Giorgio Iervasi et al., "Low-T3 syndrome," *Circulation* 107, no. 5 (2003): 708–713.

the organ. T3 binds to the heart during a heart attack and prevents it from reshaping itself unnaturally.[39,40]

Your thyroid also lowers certain inflammatory markers in your body, such as high-sensitivity C-reactive protein (hsCRP).[41] When hsCRP is elevated, cells are under duress and even dying. This leads to significant risks for heart attacks and cancer.[42,43]

On the flip side of the coin, too much thyroid is also cardiotoxic. It will burn your heart out. Having optimal thyroid levels significantly reduces these risks.

---

39. Constantinos Pantos, Iordanis Mourouzis, and Dennis V. Cokkinos, "Rebuilding the Post-infarcted Myocardium by Activating 'Physiologic' Hypertrophic Signaling Pathways: The Thyroid Hormone Paradigm," *Heart Failure Reviews* 15, no. 2 (2010): 143–154; Irwin Klein and Sara Danzi, "Thyroid Hormone Treatment to Mend a Broken Heart," *Journal of Clinical Endocrinology and Metabolism* 93, no. 4 (April 2008): 1172–1174.

40. Constantinos et al., "Thyroid Hormone and 'Cardiac Metamorphosis': Potential Therapeutic Implications," *Pharmacology and Therapeutics* 118, no. 2 (2008): 277–294.

41. Mirjam Christ-Crain et al., "Elevated C-reactive Protein and Homocysteine Values: Cardiovascular Risk Factors in Hypothyroidism? A Cross-Sectional and a Double-Blind, Placebo-Controlled Trial," *Atherosclerosis* 166, no. 2 (2003): 379–386.

42. Brian Clyne and Jonathan S. Olshaker, "The C-reactive protein," *Journal of Emergency Medicine* 17, no. 6 (1999): 1019–1025.

43. Seounghee Lee et al., "High-Sensitivity C-reactive Protein and Cancer," *Journal of Epidemiology* 21, no. 3 (2011): 161–168.

Immunological

Your thyroid is intimately linked to your immune system.

The thyroid primes and potentiates immune function.[44] If your thyroid is suboptimal, your immune system will be slow and weak. This is often triggered by stress, diet, and hormone imbalance.

As we saw in the story about Jessica, your immune system could start attacking your own thyroid. Women have a higher risk factor for this due to their higher levels of estrogen. Just like your thyroid, estrogen has a unique influence on your immune system. When it is elevated, women may develop autoimmunity.[45,46]

Having estrogen-progesterone irregularities sets an environment in which autoimmunity is more likely. Elevated estrogen also strongly reduces the bioavailability of thyroid hormone to aid with immune function.

---

44. Paolo De Vito et al., "Thyroid Hormones as Modulators of Immune Activities at the Cellular Level," *Thyroid* 21, no. 8 (2011): 879–890.

45. S. Ansar Ahmed et al., "Gender and Risk of Autoimmune Diseases: Possible Role of Estrogenic Compounds," *Environmental Health Perspectives* 107, Suppl 5 (1999): 681.

46. Maurizio Cutolo et al., "Estrogens and Autoimmune Diseases," *Annals of the New York Academy of Sciences* 1089, no. 1 (2006): 538–547.

Hepatic

It is also vital that your thyroid and liver work well together, because your liver is an important piece of the thyroid puzzle.

The precursor T4 turns into the active hormone T3 in the liver and the muscle using an enzyme called 5-prime deiodinase. That conversion is sensitive to cortisol, so if you are under severe stress, you are not going to turn T4 into T3 as well as you should.

This problem can also occur if you have a diet poor in micronutrients such as zinc and selenium. A diet high in preservatives slows down the liver's function. If your diet is full of toxins, your liver will prioritize the detoxification of your system over working with the thyroid to enhance metabolism.

Neurological

Your thyroid also affects your mental clarity.[47]

Low thyroid levels lead to poor cognitive functioning, such as weak short-term memory recall. You aren't able to juggle as many ideas at once. You may have intact memories, but you aren't able to access them as quickly as you should

---

47. F. Monzanil et al., "Subclinical Hypothyroidism: Neurobehavioral Features and Beneficial Effect of L-thyroxine Treatment," *Clinical Investigator* 71, no. 5 (1993): 367–371.

be able to.[48] If you are brainstorming and coming up with multiple ideas easily, then your thyroid is probably working well. If you try to brainstorm and can barely handle two ideas at the same time, your thyroid may be off.

Digestive

Because your thyroid controls the pace of your systems, it also directly affects your digestion.

Peristalsis is the action of your body moving food from the mouth to the colon by flexing the muscles of your intestinal tract. When you have good thyroid function, those muscles flex correctly and your body moves things through it at a healthy pace.[49]

If you don't have good thyroid function, everything slows down. You are slower to release enzymes in your pancreas. Your stomach muscles are sluggish. You're constipated.

One further thing to mention here is that balancing your thyroid is not necessarily a cure-all for weight loss. Having

---

48. Karem H. Alzoubi et al., "Levothyroxin Restores Hypothyroidism-Induced Impairment of Hippocampus-Dependent Learning and Memory: Behavioral, Electrophysiological, and Molecular Studies," *Hippocampus* 19, no. 1 (2009): 66–78.

49. Gregory L. Eastwood et al., "Reversal of Lower Esophageal Sphincter Hypotension and Esophageal Aperistalsis after Treatment for Hypothyroidism," *Journal of Clinical Gastroenterology* 4, no. 4 (1982): 307–310.

low thyroid may cause you to gain weight, but normalizing those levels only stops the increase. It does not automatically lead to weight loss. Losing weight can be one of the hardest things in the world to do. An individualized diet based on your unique metabolic needs is typically the most effective method to get rid of the extra weight and keep it off.

Just Got to Be Free

It can be difficult to get an accurate read on your thyroid levels, because some doctors may not know which tests to run.

Every hormone has a version that is free and a version that is bound. When doctors run lab work, they must include the free version of thyroid to get the most accurate picture. To ascertain thyroid levels correctly, your doctor has to measure your free T4 and free T3.

Here's where things get tricky. The liver makes proteins in your body called thyroid binding globulin. The goal of thyroid binding globulin in your body is to suck up as much thyroid hormone as it can find. Your liver uses this globulin as a way to buffer the amount of thyroid hormone in your body at any given time.

Sometimes our bodies have too much thyroid binding globulin,[50] which lessens the amount of free hormone in our

---

50. David Sarne, "Effects of the Environment, Chemicals and Drugs on Thyroid Function," (2010); K. B. Ain, Y. Mori, and

systems. So we can receive plenty of thyroid hormone, and everything can look fine when we test, but, in reality, more of the T3 and T4 is bound or inactive instead of free.

Many doctors do not run the most accurate lab tests when it comes to thyroid (the ones that test for free T3 and T4). Often, doctors select the most basic and inexpensive tests—just testing for TSH, which doesn't tell them anything useful. Some doctors make the mistake of running a total T4 or a total T3—including the bound hormones—when that is not accurate. The most accurate test measures free T3 and free T4.

It is really important to test the free versions of your thyroid hormones to get as clear a picture as possible of your thyroid health.

Diagnosis: Thyroid

Because of the complications we just discussed, it's important to acknowledge a fundamental fact of life: your doctors will probably not diagnose thyroid correctly.

Again, most doctors run only one lab, because it's cheap and easy. Almost all doctors test for TSH, which shows only

---

S. Refetoff, "Reduced Clearance of Thyroxine-Binding Globulin (TBG) with Increased Sialylation: A Mechanism for Estrogen Induced Elevation of Serum TBG Concentration," *Journal of Clinical Endocrinology and Metabolism* 65 (1987): 689–696.

what your brain thinks about how much thyroid you have. It does not test how much of the actual hormone is in your body. Even if your doctor tests beyond your TSH, he or she sometimes tests only the T4—which, remember, is inactive.

Ultimately, the only way to diagnose your thyroid is to test the free versions of your T3 and T4. Failing to get a complete picture of thyroid function results in one of the most underdiagnosed problems in women.

Here's what you need to know to get your thyroid tested correctly.

The active hormone, T3, has a reference range of 2.0 to 4.8. Typically, a woman at 2.0, the lowest end of "normal" thyroid levels, is twelve pounds heavier than a woman at the higher end of the range.[51] But everyone thrives at a different level, and no two women are exactly the same. My practice uses 3.2 as a baseline for free T3. Most women thrive when they are above this number and below 4.8.

Insurance pays the doctor the same amount of money regardless of outcome, whether he treats your thyroid or doesn't. The harm is done to *you*. That's why *you* need to understand what's really going on with your thyroid, rather than depending completely on a physician to diagnose it for you.

A thyroid disorder is not a vanity. You are not being vain if you worry about gaining weight. It is not something to be

---

51. Knudsen, "Small Differences in Thyroid Function," 4019–4024.

embarrassed about. And *you* know your body best. If something is not right, it is my job as your doctor to figure out why. We will discuss this doctor-patient relationship even more in the treatment chapter, coming up in chapter 7.

But for now, know that what you are going through is real and valid. You are sane, and you are strong. And, with some adjustments, you are going to be all right.

My Theory

I have a theory about the thyroid based on my education and observation of thousands of patients over the years. I believe that, evolutionarily speaking, our thyroids are programmed to start lowering as we age.

It is a fact that people's thyroids start to be less active as they get older. Our brains send fewer signals for thyroid hormone production.

I personally think this is an evolutionary trait. If our metabolisms slow down, we eat less food. And we use fewer resources from the community, which can then be used for younger people. Our ancestors slowed their physical activity in their forties and fifties.

The problem in modern times, of course, is that we are now more active throughout our lifespans than we ever have been. And stress levels aren't decreasing as we age. It is common for people in their sixties to still be working full time. Our ancestors didn't even live to be sixty, much less work or do anything constructive. So biologically, we are wired to start winding down at an age at which we still expect to have decades longer of productive living.

In my mind, this only serves to highlight the importance of taking care of your thyroid and managing any issues as early as possible. Doing so not only improves your metabolism in the present but also helps to ensure that you can stay as active as possible, as long as possible. And that is an empowered life!

You have now learned about your body and mind, your female hormones, and the thermostat for your metabolism. But what else makes up the balance of our bodies and hormones? Testosterone is a critical piece of hormone balance for both women and men, as we'll discuss in chapter 5.

Testosterone

The Plan

In late 2008, I met with a husband and wife who came to see me together. Whenever a husband brings his wife in, it can go one of two ways. The first way? He genuinely loves his wife and wants to help her and advocate for her. The second? It can be a little more selfish.

This particular visit went the second way.

Mark made an appointment for his wife, Francine, because he had heard that testosterone could improve a woman's libido. Next to him, Francine was timid and quiet, not making eye contact or speaking much. When I ran some tests, the results showed that Francine's testosterone levels were in fact low. So she agreed to start testosterone therapy.

Right away, Francine responded well to therapy and regained her libido. But that wasn't the only improvement.

Within the first month, Mark called me up and demanded, "What are you doing with my wife? She's no longer following the plan!" He sounded like a controlling eight-year-old, and no wonder: it seemed that Francine was no longer playing by his domineering rules.

I was able to talk to Francine on her own, because she stopped bringing Mark to her appointments. She told me, "Yeah, I have a libido, but I also have so much baggage with this man. He was so controlling of me, and I never felt heard!" So she stood up to him. She had never done that before.

Shortly after that conversation, she decided to choose her own happiness. She left him. Because you know what? She had a plan of her own, for her own life, of what she wanted to do—a plan she had been unable to see clearly before.

Balancing Francine's testosterone gave her just the courage and confidence she needed to start living life on her own terms. That is the power of testosterone in regaining hormone balance.

Testosterone: Not Just for Men

I mentioned this previously, but it bears repeating: women are supposed to have some testosterone in their bodies. Just as men produce estrogen, women's bodies also produce testosterone.[52]

Testosterone is a hormone produced in low amounts in your ovaries and adrenal glands. Its role in your body is to modulate the growth effect of estrogen, ensure the production

---

52. H. S. Kaplan and T. Owett, "The Female Androgen Deficiency Syndrome," *Journal of Sex and Marital Therapy* 19 (1993): 3–24.

of healthy skeletal and cardiac muscle, regulate bone density, and help modulate brain chemistry.[53,54,55,56,57,58,59,60]

53. N. B. Watts et al., "Comparison of Oral Estrogens and Estrogens Plus Androgen on Bone Mineral Density, Menopausal Symptoms, and Lipid-Lipoprotein Profiles in Surgical Menopause," *Obstetrics and Gynecology* 85 (1995): 529–537 [published correction appears in *Obstetrics and Gynecology* 85, no. 5 pt 1 (1995): 668].

54. E. Barrett-Connor et al., "A Two-Year, Double-Blind Comparison of Estrogen-Androgen and Conjugated Estrogens in Surgically Menopausal Women: Effects on Bone Mineral Density, Symptoms and Lipid Profiles," *Journal of Reproductive Medicine* 44 (1999):1012–1020.

55. N. L. McCoy and J. M. Davidson, "A Longitudinal Study of the Effects of Menopause on Sexuality," *Maturitas* 7 (1985): 203–210.

56. S. R. Davis et al., "Testosterone Enhances Estradiol's Effects on Postmenopausal Bone Density and Sexuality," *Maturitas* 21 (1995): 227–236.

57. R. A. Lobo et al., "Comparative Effects of Oral Esterified Estrogens with and without Methyltestosterone on Endocrine Profiles and Dimensions of Sexual Function in Postmenopausal Women with Hypoactive Sexual Desire," *Fertility and Sterility* 79 (2003): 1341–1352.

58. P. Sarrel, B. Dobay, and B. Wiita, "Estrogen and Estrogen-Androgen Replacement in Postmenopausal Women Dissatisfied with Estrogen-Only Therapy: Sexual Behavior and Neuroendocrine Responses," *Journal of Reproductive Medicine* 43 (1998): 847–856.

59. H. Burger et al., "Effect of Combined Implants of Testradiol and Testosterone on Libido in Postmenopausal Women," *British Medical Journal* 294 (1987): 936–937.

60. J. L Shifren et al., "Transdermal Testosterone Treatment in Women with Impaired Sexual Function after Oophorectomy," *New England Journal of Medicine* 343 (2000): 682–688.

Testosterone is active in the parts of the brain associated with confidence, assertiveness, and boundary setting. And in that part of the brain are the deep centers of drive—also called the limbic system. This cone-shaped part of your brain houses the aggressive part of you—the part that takes risk.[61] It's a part of you that is territorial and tribal. It's also associated with sexual interest,[62] drive, memory improvement,[63,64] and ambition.[65]

61. Steven J. Stanton, Scott H. Liening, and Oliver C. Schultheiss, "Testosterone Is Positively Associated with Risktaking in the Iowa Gambling Task," *Hormones and Behavior* 59, no. 2 (2011): 252–256.

62. Katherine L. Goldey and Sari M. van Anders, "Sexy Thoughts: Effects of Sexual Cognitions on Testosterone, Cortisol, and Arousal in Women," *Hormones and Behavior* 59, no. 5 (2011): 754–764.

63. O. T. Wolf and C. Kirschbaum, "Endogenous Estradiol and Testosterone Levels Are Associated with Cognitive Performance in Older Women and Men," *Hormones and Behavior* 41 (2002): 259–266.

64. Jianxin Jia et al., "Amelioratory Effects of Testosterone Treatment on Cognitive Performance Deficits Induced by Soluble Aβ1–42 Oligomers Injected into the Hippocampus," *Hormones and Behavior* 64, no. 3 (2013): 477–486.

65. Paola Sapienza, Luigi Zingales, and Dario Maestripieri, "Gender Differences in Financial Risk Aversion and Career Choices Are Affected by Testosterone," *Proceedings of the National Academy of Sciences* 106, no. 36 (2009): 15268–15273.

When you have healthy testosterone levels, those traits become part of your life and the way you act in the world. If you don't have the correct level of testosterone, all of those important things just drop off.

Unfortunately, it is a common occurrence in America these days for testosterone levels to be low, in both men and women.

Plastics play a role in this lower production of testosterone. Phthalates[66] and BPA, present in many plastics until fairly recently, have been shown to cause permanent damage to endocrine cells and their production of testosterone.

Women experience a steady decline in testosterone levels from their twenties to menopause. No clear lower limit exists as an established norm for testosterone levels in women.[67] This is because, unfortunately, research regarding women and hormones—particularly testosterone—is scant. Other than the research that shows plastics cut down testosterone production and oral contraceptives reduce testosterone levels, we just don't have a profound amount of research explaining

---

66. John D. Meeker and Kelly K. Ferguson, "Urinary Phthalate Metabolites Are Associated with Decreased Serum Testosterone in Men, Women, and Children from NHANES 2011–2012," *Journal of Clinical Endocrinology and Metabolism* 99, no. 11 (2014): 4346–4352.

67. Katherine Margo and Robert Winn, "Testosterone Treatments: Why, When, and How," *American Family Physician* 73, no. 9 (2006): 1591–1598.

why it drops so low. Nevertheless, there's no denying the important role testosterone plays in a rich, fulfilling life.

The frontal cortex of your brain, the psychological part associated with personality and consciousness, comprises all the experiences you have had in your life.

I like to think of the brain's frontal cortex as a lens. In a grown woman, that lens is thick; women develop their cortexes faster because they mature faster. And that lens is colored with all the beautiful things in your life: whom you've become as a woman, your friendships, your beliefs, all the things you love in life. It is like a stained-glass window of life experiences.

The biological limbic system is the light behind that lens, and hormones such as testosterone affect the brightness of that light.

Balancing this hormone turns up the light so you can shine just right, neither too dim nor too bright.

In this chapter, we will examine testosterone's purposes in the body—yes, including its role in treating libido—and the potential side effects of testosterone therapy.

Beyond Libido

Everyone thinks testosterone is just for libido. But that same deep part of the brain where libido lives, which gets stimulated by testosterone, also contains confidence, assertiveness, and aggressiveness.

These traits tend to be socially attributed to men, but it is essential for women to have a healthy expression of these qualities as well.

People with healthy testosterone levels are better entrepreneurs.[68] They are better salespeople. They take more risks in their careers and set more emotional boundaries.[69] You are not a healthy woman without those traits. And that is just part of why you need testosterone as much as men do, but at a level specific to your personal chemistry.

Testosterone is also widely accepted for its ability to prevent depression and to improve mental well-being in women.[70] It also helps to increase bone density[71,72] and build muscle. Some of the early uses of testosterone in women include using it to treat severe breast pain and PMS.

_____

68. Roderick E. White, Stewart Thornhill, and Elizabeth Hampson, "Entrepreneurs and Evolutionary Biology: The Relationship between Testosterone and New Venture Creation," *Organizational Behavior and Human Decision Processes* 100, no. 1 (2006): 21–34.

69. Elizabeth Cashdan, "Hormones and Competitive Aggression in Women," *Aggressive Behavior* 29, no. 2 (2003): 107–115.

70. B. B. Sherwin, "Affective Changes with Estrogen and Androgen Replacement Therapy in Surgically Menopausal Women," *Journal of Affective Disorders* 14 (1988): 177–187.

71. N. B. Watts, "Comparison of Oral Estrogens," 529–537.

72. E. Barrett-Connor, "A Two-Year, Double-Blind Comparison," 1012–1020.

Ultimately, I believe testosterone's goal is to be a subordinate to progesterone. In my professional medical opinion, testosterone should not be used as a stand-alone therapy in a woman, but rather in balance alongside estrogen and progesterone.

Testosterone therapy's primary function is to support progesterone's estrogen-balancing function. If your estrogen and progesterone are fine, your testosterone levels are probably in balance, too. If your estrogen and progesterone levels are off, your testosterone probably is too. It is best to treat them together, although I always look to progesterone first.

Although easily forgotten about as a hormone in women, testosterone is a really important aspect of everyone's central drive. When your testosterone level is healthy, your brain chemistry is rounded out with this whole new dimension of your personality.

But Sometimes It Is about Sex

Now, testosterone is not *just* about libido, but by helping to awaken that part of your brain, it does work amazingly to improve libido in women.

If you have no testosterone, you will have markedly decreased sexual desire and absent or markedly decreased orgasms. For a doctor to ignore this issue is profoundly disrespectful to you as a woman—to all women—and is a disservice to your sexuality. If, however, your testosterone levels are normalized, and you feel healthy and safe, you can have a whole sexual revolution of yourself and that erotic part of your identity. This is a beautiful aspect of testosterone's effect, but it is important to remember that it is not the only part.

Remember the image of the projector? Part of your cortex—the lens—is associated with libido. It is possible for the lens to be damaged. A woman could have had a sexual trauma that affects her libido, for example. No amount of hormone can fix that.

However, in many cases, the problem resides in the limbic system. In other words, the problem may be with the light, not the lens. And the light can be adjusted using testosterone. If the real cause of the issue is the light, it is not fair *to you* that society blames the lens.

Too many books, movies, and TV shows place the blame for low libido on women, making it seem like a conscious choice. The stereotype of a woman repulsed by the idea of sex has been a severe disservice to women. It affects not only your self-esteem, but also your identity. Of course, that stereotype is going to make you feel guilty that your libido has diminished, and that is not okay. Low libido can have a psychological cause or a biological cause, and this fact deserves to be acknowledged.

Fortunately, when the problem lies in the limbic system, it is biological in nature, so we can treat that. The solution for low testosterone tied to the limbic system is simpler than when it is tied to the cortex, which is psychological. If the limbic system has no testosterone, the hormone can be replaced.

I'm not trying to write a book about sex, but sex is an important part of life. And you deserve to have that part be active and robust. You deserve a completely fulfilling life.

Put It in Reverse

Let me tell you the truth about testosterone therapy. Balancing a woman's testosterone is a very precise process.

My goal as a physician is to adjust your body's hormones to be at the right level. With hormone replacement therapy, I can get your testosterone within the "normal" range. But even though the imbalance can be corrected to look good on your lab results, it's not as good as it would be if your ovaries were producing the hormone themselves. Testosterone supplementation is a temperamental process requiring a lot of medical experience and consistent oversight during treatment.

The bright side is that the dose range we use in women is so low that the chance for side effects is minimal. With these doses, any adverse side effects are completely reversible.

When a woman's body makes testosterone, it constantly secretes from the ovaries and adrenal glands in tiny increments at a controlled rate of release. But when I give a woman an injection of testosterone, I have to give her about a week's worth at once. It is critical to get the dose right so the body can handle the amount provided in a healthy fashion.

You have to be very proactive with the management of testosterone and stay current on lab work to help avoid side effects.

Testosterone has four benefits that can sometimes turn into side effects: increased head hair in women,[73] which can lead to increased body hair; increased skin moisture, which can lead to breakouts; heightened libido when first treated, which is usually temporary; and increased sensitivity of the clitoris. If any of these increases too much, we lower the dose. Most side effects diminish or disappear in a month, but if not, we continue to adjust the dose.

The body was made naturally as a masterpiece, like the Sistine Chapel. The human body is a precise, beautiful work of art. And going in there to do testosterone replacement is almost like an eight-year-old with finger paints trying to fix a broken piece of the painting. I'll use labs, and I'll come close, and I will always do my best. But treatment will never recreate the original masterpiece.

I would rather try to patch that piece than leave it broken, though. To me, the most important aspect of treating a

---

73. R. L. Glaser, C. Dimitrakakis, and A. G. Messenger, "Improvement in Scalp Hair Growth in Androgen-Deficient Women Treated with Testosterone: A Questionnaire Study," *British Journal of Dermatology* 166, no. 2 (2012): 274–278.

woman is seeing her as a whole human being. Testosterone plays a vital role in being a complete woman.

Stand Up for Yourself

One of my favorite stories is of a woman named Tracy, whom I treated with testosterone therapy.

Tracy worked in a hostile workplace, selling homeowner's insurance in a high-stress environment.

She came back to see me a few weeks after we started her on the hormones, and she was upset. "You've got to get this stuff out of me," she pleaded. "You've got to stop this!"

Completely baffled, I asked her, "What?"

Very seriously, she looked at me and said, "I'm turning into a bitch."

She explained that, in the past, whenever her boss was mean or yelled at her, she would just take it. But this time, when he yelled at her, she stood up for herself.

And she wasn't used to that new mood swing in the other direction.

But it didn't take Tracy long to realize that she was not being a bitch. She was asserting her feelings and setting boundaries. Her boss had tried to reframe that and portray her behavior in a stereotypical way. Tracy stood her ground and stood up for herself. She stayed in that work environment for a while, cautiously trying out her new voice. Over time, the hostile atmosphere stopped taking such a huge emotional toll on her. Her boss's attempts to bully her were met with a confident "No." At the end of each day, Tracy left work feeling good about herself.

And that confidence made all the difference in her life.

At this point, you have learned all about the hormones that affect your body and mind. But what happens when your hormones are in balance and you *still* don't feel right? That's when it's time to take a closer look at what's happening inside your brain. In the next chapter, we will cover neurotransmitters.

Chapter 6

Neurotransmitters

Picture Perfect

Picture the absolute perfect moment in life, that moment when all the stars are aligned and you feel your best emotionally, physically, and spiritually.

Imagine that everything in your life is good. You have all the relationships you want around you. You bask in the love and support of your family, wonderful friends who cherish you, and the intimate relationship you have always desired. Your job is satisfying and fulfilling. Your dream to have everything that makes you happy is not a dream; it's real.

You are in harmony with your life.

You place value in yourself, and you know that you worked really hard to become the person you are today. You have gratitude for the people who have come into your life and share it with you. You are thankful for all you have.

Picture this perfect life. Then imagine removing your ability to feel the joy and satisfaction that such a life would bring. The circumstances are still the same, but now you swing toward feeling sad all the time, as if all the happiness has been removed from your life.

This is what it feels like when you have an imbalance in your neurotransmitters.

On top of feeling this way, people in your life start telling you, "I don't understand why you're so upset. I don't know why you're so sad. Everything in your life is good. You should just snap out of it!"

But you can't. Logically, you see how your experience of life is not consistent with your emotional state. But logic won't put the joy back into a beautiful sunset or a romantic dinner. This disconnect begins with a chemical problem in your brain.

But here's the good news: just like hormone imbalance, this problem in your brain can be corrected.

Transmission Disruption

If you want to be happy but have an impending sense that something's going to go wrong any minute, you may have a neurotransmitter defect.

Neurotransmitters are the chemical packets sent by your brain from neuron to neuron to stimulate emotional status. Many neurotransmitters start off as proteins in your diet. As you consume the protein, it breaks down into peptides in the stomach and absorbs into the bloodstream. From there, the peptides find their way to neurons, which convert them into neurotransmitters using enzymes that are modulated by hormones.

When your neurotransmitters are functioning properly, you are able to see that life is good. But when they are not, your life can be profoundly affected. If you're not producing serotonin, it's difficult to feel happiness. If you're not producing GABA, you're going to feel anxious. If you're not producing melatonin, you're not going to sleep. And if your dopamine—the reward center of the brain—is off, you're going to feel lost and depressed.

If you have a neurotransmitter imbalance, you feel depleted, deprived, and diminished. In fact, any time a patient comes in with emotional symptoms, I look to neurotransmitters immediately.

When I triage a patient, the very first thing I consider is her emotional state. Then I think about which neurotransmitters may be involved with those emotions and which hormones trigger those neurotransmitters. Then I try to find the connection.

More often than not, a hormone imbalance has created a neurotransmitter imbalance.

In those cases, we go after the cause: the hormone. Once we address the hormone imbalance, the neurotransmitter production can go back online. In some cases, the neurotransmitter imbalance is so severe that it causes significant emotional instability. In those cases, it would take too long for the hormones to balance out and offer some relief, so I treat the neurotransmitters directly.

No matter what, you are the priority. The most important thing is for you to experience your life as a sane, healthy woman and to appreciate how beautiful it is.

In this chapter, we are going to look at the role of stress and vitamins in neurotransmitter production, the methods for directly treating any imbalances, and neurotransmitter issues that are not caused by hormones.

Cooking Up Neurotransmitters

What affects neurotransmitter production in the body?

Nutrition, hormones, and stress all affect your body's production of neurotransmitters, whether positively or negatively. As we talked about earlier, sustained, chronic stress elevates cortisol in your body. That chronic cortisol release inhibits the production of serotonin and many other neurotransmitters in your brain.

When this happens, a supplement called 5-hydroxytryptophan (5-HTP), the immediate precursor to serotonin, will help restore short-term balance. To truly treat the imbalance, however, you have to address the root cause: stress. You have to get out of the war zone, so to speak, or use therapy to figure out the underlying cause of a traumatic response you may be experiencing. Until that happens, the neurotransmitter issue itself will not be fixed.

Stress is not the only factor in imbalanced neurotransmitter production. If hormones are one factor for the production of neurotransmitters, then proper nutrition is the cofactor. That includes getting enough vitamins in your diet.

For example, vitamin B6 is the single most important vitamin to help your body turn the food you eat into neurotransmitters. B6 is especially important when it comes to making dopamine, the neurotransmitter of reward and pleasure. Similarly, to make serotonin—the neurotransmitter of balance and happiness—you need folate, zinc, and—you guessed it—more vitamin B6.

The metabolism of estrogen, more than any other hormone in your body, uses up vitamin B6. If you have a lot of estrogen, your liver will require a significant amount of B6 to process and metabolize it. When that happens, you don't have any vitamin B6 left to generate the necessary neurotransmitters for your brain.

Neurotransmitters can be thrown off balance by hormone imbalances, as well as by nutritional deficiencies. Vitamins are necessary for neurotransmitter and hormone production. Vitamin deficiencies are a double whammy to your system. When the individual ingredients are balanced, they work in harmony. But when one level is thrown off, it can derail everything.

So how can you treat this imbalance on every level?

You begin by looking at what a given vitamin supports in your body. If a woman presents with a lot of estrogen, low serotonin, and signs of a neurotransmitter imbalance, I will give her vitamin B6 because I know it will help to support those symptoms. However, the B6 supplement is a temporary solution. To address the long-term issue, we will look at her diet to make sure her nutritional intake of B6 is optimal.

Vitamin B12 and folic acid are also essential for neurotransmitter synthesis. Deficiencies of either vitamin are even easier to treat by looking for the downstream metabolites. One of the ways to know B12 and folic acid are doing their jobs is if your cells are duplicating at a healthy pace. To test this pathway, your doctor will run a lab called mean corpuscular volume, or MCV. If it comes back elevated, in most cases it will be because of a B12 and/or folic acid deficiency.

Proper nutrition is vitally important to your health. Without it, your body cannot convert food into neurotransmitters the way it needs to. And your diet is the ideal source of nutrition. Diets chronically deficient in protein, vitamins, minerals, and antioxidants play a role in neurotransmitter deficiencies. Making sure you eat a balanced diet is an essential part of treating your whole person.

Treating Neurotransmitters

Neurotransmitter defects can be tested and directly treated. You do not always have to use prescriptions such as antidepressants. Often, it can be just as effective to use the direct precursor to the neurotransmitter to restore balance in this area.

When I talk about "the direct precursor," I'm referring to the protein or peptide that generates a particular neurotransmitter.

For example, as we've discussed, serotonin is created by its precursor, 5-HTP. To treat depression from serotonin deficiency, I give the patient 5-HTP. That's all there is to this treatment, other than checking labs to confirm that the dose is correct.

Anxiety due to GABA deficiency can also be treated with the precursors to GABA, though this one is a little more complex. In this case, glutamine turns into glutamic acid, which then turns into GABA. However, giving someone glutamine doesn't always work. You can also give GABA itself as a supplement, but that doesn't always cross over and work as well as it could.

Therefore, when GABA levels measure low on lab work and the patient presents with anxiety, I will use a natural GABA substitute. This is called 5-amino-4-phenylbutyric acid, and it binds to the GABA receptor really well. Using this derivative helps to calm down the brain chemistry and normalize it.

Treating a melatonin deficiency is the simplest of all. There aren't even any precursors involved. You just take melatonin itself until the serotonin levels are optimized and you can sleep well again.

Neurotransmitters generally don't cause side effects, making them a safe method for restoring balance to your body.

What If It's Not Hormones?

Though hormone imbalance is most often the trigger of an issue with neurotransmitters, that is not always the case. Once we have either determined that your hormones are fine or found and treated any imbalances there, I jump up to neurotransmitter treatment.

For some people, the problems occur due to aging or a genetic irregularity that affects their ability to create neurotransmitters.

One example of a genetic irregularity is methylenetetra-hydrofolate reductase deficiency, or MTHFR, which means that dietary folic acid is unable to be converted into its active version, methyl folate. This irregularity can cause a number of health problems, including risk factors for heart attacks and issues with brain chemistry. If you don't have methyl folic acid, you don't make serotonin. And no serotonin means no melatonin.

Other people's systems genetically don't turn serotonin into melatonin very well because they have a slow enzyme pathway. Enzyme pathways also slow down as we age. And if an enzyme pathway slows down too much, it shuts off.

The good news is that many genetic irregularities can be tested for and effectively treated.

I use targeted amino acid therapy to balance neurotransmitters. Instead of giving a patient a drug such as Xanax or Valium that artificially binds to the GABA receptor, we target the amino acid that is deficient. For example, as mentioned previously, for a serotonin deficiency, I prescribe the patient the amino acid 5-HTP.

This method of therapy has proven to be very safe, verifiable, and incredibly simple, like putting gasoline in your car when the gas gauge is low. Once your tank is full, you can drive anywhere you want to go.

Your Own Rhythm

Even with as many patients as I see, sometimes someone will remind me of something basic I've forgotten. One of my patients, James, recently reminded me that men have neurotransmitter defects just as women do.

James came in with chronic headaches. While I know that a serotonin deficiency can trigger headaches, that's not always the first thing I go to with male patients. So I had James try an elimination diet, removing possible triggers such as gluten and dairy. Magnesium citrate has often helped me treat chronic headaches. In James's case, however, it did not help, even with intravenous infusions. Nothing worked to get his headaches under control.

Finally, on his fourth visit, I tested his neurotransmitters. Sure enough, James had a serotonin deficiency.

James was not depressed, even though serotonin deficiency is most often associated with depression. But this imbalance was causing his headaches, which is a less common side effect of low serotonin. Ironically, the triptan class of medication, such as sumatriptan, stops headaches by targeting serotonin.

I prescribed James 5-HTP, and the headaches went away. Best of all, unlike the prescription medications, the treatment was safe and healthy. He experienced no side effects.

The best treatments out there look to the whole person and work to restore balance as effectively and safely as possible. This is true for hormones as well as neurotransmitters.

You now have looked at several different causes of imbalance in your body. But how can you know which to treat, which treatment is best, and how to ask your doctor for help? The next chapter discusses how to get treatment, and it will help you answer those questions.

Chapter 7

Treatment

A New Flute

In the early 1990s, I spent two years studying Baroque flute making with renowned flute maker Patrick Olwell. He was a mentor who taught me not only to see each handmade flute as a work of art, but also to view each patient as unique. His influence on me can be felt every day in the treatment room.

I see women's health as a handmade instrument requiring focus and precision.

Patrick acquires beautiful wood from all over the world, each piece completely different from the next. Different trees have different densities and different amounts of water; they have received different amounts of sunlight and elements from the soil. Even two pieces of wood from the same tree can sound completely different.

The same thing is true with women: no two are completely the same.

Not every woman is going to need treatment using progesterone. It won't always be estrogen, or testosterone, or thyroid. Nutrients won't be the solution for every woman, and two women with the same condition may respond to two completely different treatments, each in her own unique way.

One of the first things I learned when I started practicing medicine was never to make the mistake of believing that what worked for one person would work for the next.

When I meet you as a new patient, I view the experience like playing a new flute for the first time. I want to know what may be out of tune and how to get it to work correctly. I want to know *why* your unique symptoms are affecting you the way they are. And I want to know how all the pieces work together in harmony.

Because when you play it perfectly, a new flute has a beauty all its own.

Two-Pronged Approach to Treatment

I define treatment differently from how many other physicians do.

If you go into your doctor's office with something as simple as depression, your doctor will generally just prescribe an antidepressant medication. That doctor's goal is to stabilize you on that specific medication. And this can be a noble goal to give you back your life.

But I don't think this should be the endgame for a physician.

Stabilizing a patient should, of course, be the first step of a physician's plan. But stopping at stabilizing the patient doesn't address what's really wrong. More than that, your doctor should *want* to figure out why you are having this specific problem. And upon figuring that out, the doctor should exercise every effort at his or her disposal to solve it. If the problem can't be solved completely, a doctor should make the treatment as precise and effective as possible, with the fewest side effects.

I see treatment as a commitment to each patient to do your absolute best.

Committing to that level of treatment should be part of your calling as a doctor. If it's not your calling, or you don't give it everything you can, you may harm the patient. But if you do your best with all the research and resources available to you, then you are going to do good work in this world. You will start to change lives.

As a patient, and as a person, when you have a really good doctor, you have someone who cares about you. This person is your advocate, always in your corner. And this relationship will be obvious. You will be able to see and feel his or her empathy. You will know that your doctor cares and wants to figure this out with you. Not only will your doctor do his or her best, but that person will want you to be the best *you* that you can be.

Treatment, in my mind, covers two aspects, which we are going to discuss in this chapter: the actual treatment you need for the hormonal or neurotransmitter imbalances previously discussed, and the way in which you communicate with your doctor to get what you need in terms of treatment. Both are necessary for you to become a full advocate for your own health.

Let's Talk Treatments

In each of the previous chapters, we discussed potential imbalances and some of their treatments. Now, we're going to break it down even further.

For each of the categories covered in the previous chapters, I am going to explain how to talk to your doctor about the issue and exactly what treatments you want to ask about.

Adrenals

If you feel that your symptoms are connected to a lot of stress in your life, you will want to get your adrenal glands tested.

To see the most accurate picture of your adrenal glands, you want to run cortisol tests four times during the day: when you first wake up, mid-morning, midday, and mid-evening. That way, we can see how cortisol moves through the body with your circadian rhythm. It is normal for cortisol to start high in the morning and begin to drop as the day goes on.

When we test cortisol more than once in the same day, we can see if there are unexpected increases. This indicates that the adrenal gland is being stimulated by the fight-or-flight hormones epinephrine and norepinephrine, which cause a spike in cortisol and are indicative of stressful conditions.

Labbing cortisol four times during the day gives us a lot of information to evaluate your level of stress.

Stress has four causes: physical stress, such as overwork or poor sleep; chemical stress, such as food allergies or hormone imbalance; thermal stress, such as overheating or overchilling the body; and emotional, or mental, stress.

Stress occurs in three stages. In stage one, the alarm phase, you are reacting to a new and immediate stressor. You feel alert, because your body has higher levels of epinephrine and norepinephrine. This causes your heart to beat faster, your breathing to speed up, and your muscles to tense. Your attention narrows, and you focus mainly on the stressor. The alarm phase, also called the fight-or-flight response, is meant to keep you alive in a stressful situation.

In the second stage, called the resistance phase, the stress has gone from temporary to long term. In cases like this, the stressor can be a hostile workplace, a spouse you do not feel connected to, or the loss of a loved one. During the resistance phase, the body tries to shore up and resist the stressor. Common symptoms include the restless feelings from the alarm phase, sugar cravings, and weight gain from increased cortisol. Elevated cortisol also weakens the immune system, opening the door to illness.

Finally, stage three is the exhaustion phase, during which the body just gives up. If your adrenals have been releasing cortisol and epinephrine day after day, and your nervous system has been releasing norepinephrine, sooner or later your body will wear out. At this point of total burnout, your system has no more cortisol, epinephrine, or norepinephrine—just exhaustion.

Treating stress is not easy. It can call for making some hard decisions, including lifestyle changes to relieve the pressure stress puts on your body.

Short-term stress is not always a medical issue. And research shows that women respond very differently to stress than men do. Men in acute stress tend to really live up to "fight or flight." Women may instead respond with the need to nurture and bond. This response is termed "tend and befriend."[74]

When my wife is stressed, she wants to ensure the house is in order and to spend time with our children. This is her way of tending. She also wants to discuss her stress with me, not so I can fix it, but so she can share her feelings with me, which is part of befriending.

---

74. Shelley E. Taylor et al., "Biobehavioral Responses to Stress in Females: Tend-and-Befriend, Not Fight-or-Flight," *Psychological Review* 107, no. 3 (July 2000): 411–429.

Men approach stress relief very differently. It took me years to understand that my wife does not require a solution; she is more than capable of providing that for herself. What she needs is for me to hear her, to understand her, and to support her.

That balance at home, along with a solid support network, will help you manage short-term stress in your life as well.

If the stress looks like it will be long term, you may have to ask yourself, "Is the stress worth it? How will I be able to overcome this stress?" You will still need the support system we discussed above, but you may need medical support as well.

You and your doctor will need to discuss your options. It is important that you are empowered to make the healthy decisions you need to make. No matter what, this is the time when it is critical for your doctor to create a healthy line of judgment-free communication. You and your doctor can work together to come up with a plan to help sustain your biological health.

During this time, we look at neurotransmitters, cortisol, and blood sugar. If your neurotransmitters are out of balance, commonly seen as elevated epinephrine and norepinephrine with low GABA and serotonin, you will experience stress at a higher level. It is important to balance your brain chemistry as part of balancing and treating your adrenals. Your cortisol and blood sugar may also be elevated, so we work on lowering cortisol and adjusting your diet to reduce blood sugar levels.

If long-term stress has not been managed, you may see your doctor only after your system has finally broken down and you've hit the exhaustion phase. Lab work would show depleted cortisol and adrenaline. Treatment is intensive for this. Optimization of diet, hormones, sleep, and recreation is essential, as is the management of blood sugar, cholesterol, and neurotransmitters. Your doctor may also want to add the direct supplementation of cortisol.

Cortisol is a difficult hormone to work with; it is temperamental. If the dose is too low, you feel no difference; if it is too high, you feel anxious and depressed. I cannot overstate how important it is to retest cortisol regularly to monitor the dose and lower it as the body recovers.

A lot can go wrong during stage three, including heart attack, type 2 diabetes, and obesity. You will need a doctor dedicated to running the necessary labs and prescribing medication precisely.

Estrogen and Progesterone

If you have symptoms that shift throughout the month, associated with your menstrual cycle, such as PMS, premenstrual dysphoric disorder (PMDD), or perimenopausal symptoms, you need to say to your doctor, "I believe I have a hormone-related problem." And then you should ask for lab work to be run.

Progesterone and estrogen should never be tested at a random time. Health cannot be measured by a single snapshot; rather, you need a portrait of the dynamic flow of your body. In this case, your hormones need to be labbed during the luteal phase of your cycle, typically day twenty-one of a twenty-eight-day cycle.

If your cycle is shorter or longer, your doctor will need to adjust the date. If your cycle is too long, chances are you have low progesterone. Estrogen has been stimulating the lining of the uterus, and after a while, it can't support that tissue anymore, so it releases it. If your cycle is too short, it is normally due to low estrogen.

Ask your doctor to test progesterone and estrogen on day twenty-one. At that time, you should run other labs important to show you the big picture, possibly including estradiol, testosterone, and thyroid. These basic tests will show you where your cycle is and tell you whether you are too high in estrogen or too low in progesterone. It is essential that your doctor get to the bottom of why you may not have enough progesterone.

As we discussed in chapter 3, supplementing with natural progesterone can correct your imbalance.

Some physicians like to prescribe topical progesterone. I would warn you not to use this medication, because topical hormones will spread to your partner, your children,[75,76] and even your pets.[77] The FDA has released numerous warnings over the years regarding the use of topical hormones.

Thyroid

If, after reading the chapter on thyroid, you believe you have a hypothyroid issue, the first step is to see your physician and ask him or her to run a thyroid panel. The most basic thyroid panel should include TSH, free T3, and free T4. If you are under chronic stress, you should also add something called reverse T3. You should feel comfortable requesting an autoimmune thyroid panel as well.

We discussed TSH, free T3, and free T4 in chapter 4. Under times of stress or malnutrition, your body will sometimes make a substance called reverse T3. This is a hormone

75. E. I. Felner and P. C. White, "Prepubertal Gynecomastia: Indirect Exposure to Estrogen Cream," *Pediatrics* (2000), accessed July 6, 2010. http://www.pediatrics.org/cgi/content/full/105/4/e55.

76. C. V. DiRaimondo, A. C. Roach, and C. K. Meador, "Gynecomastia from Exposure to Vaginal Estrogen Cream," *New England Journal of Medicine* 302 (1980): 1089–1090.

77. E. Lau, "Hormone Replacement Skin Products Affect Users' Pets, Confound Veterinarians," http://news.vin.com/VINNews.aspx?articleId=15950.

that looks like T3, but it doesn't have a biological function. Worse, it blocks real T3 from working.

Normally, when your T4 turns into T3, it uses an enzyme called 5 prime deiodinase. But if you're under stress, or if you have nutritional deficiencies, cortisol will change that enzyme into 5 deiodinase, which is not prime. Reverse T3 blocks the receptors on your cells so that they can't be activated by normal T3. This blockage causes your metabolism to shut down. The issue can be addressed by treating cortisol levels and making sure you are not malnourished, which can be tested via a blood panel.

If your doctor runs your basic thyroid panel and the levels look optimal, but you still feel run down, ask to have your reverse T3 tested as well. This is also the time to check for an autoimmune thyroid issue, which should be screened in every woman presenting with thyroid issues.

Although not very useful in diagnosis, TSH shouldn't be ignored. If TSH is low, your pituitary believes you have plenty of thyroid hormone. If it is high, then it means your pituitary believes you have too little thyroid hormone.

Free T4 can be helpful in knowing how healthy your thyroid gland is. If it is low, your thyroid gland itself may be the cause of your low thyroid.

Free T3 is the single most important lab you can use. It is essential for your physician to work to get your T3 to rest at an optimal level.

Your doctor may try to put you on a stand-alone T4 therapy using Synthroid or levothyroxine. These are not bad medications, but they are not complete, and they do not work well on their own. Giving T3 and T4 together is a better degree of care. I primarily use Nature-Throid in my practice. Made of T4 and T3 in a natural, biologic ratio, Nature-Throid is incredibly inexpensive and can be found in almost any pharmacy in the country.

Testosterone

Testosterone can be tested any time of the month.

Just as with thyroid, you have both free testosterone and bound testosterone, which is bound to sex hormone binding globulin. Besides being ineffective, bound testosterone is also inert. Therefore, you should ask your doctor to test your free testosterone, the most important marker for healthy testosterone levels. Even though free testosterone is so crucial, most doctors do not run this lab.

Not every lab company runs the same free testosterone lab, and some labs yield better-quality results than others. I have had a lot of success using Access Medical Labs in Jupiter, Florida, for this test. I find that women respond best when free testosterone is in the fiftieth to sixtieth percentile.

The journal *American Family Physician* advocates giving women testosterone without testing first because it claims that testosterone levels will always appear elevated in a woman.[78] I do not agree with this. Although your total testosterone levels may look elevated, it doesn't give you a clear picture of your bioavailable testosterone levels.[79,80] Measuring free testosterone is a key indicator of how well treatment is working in your body. This alone is an important reason to test it.

Most endocrinologists also advocate a once-a-month injection for testosterone treatment in women,[81] but I do not agree with this, either. I believe you need to mimic the natural release of testosterone in your body as much as possible, which is better done with a weekly injection. When you approach treatment this way, your dosage of testosterone can be reduced, and the side effects can be minimized.

I strongly recommend against topical testosterone. As with topical progesterone, testosterone creams and ointments are known to spread to the people around you. For more information on safe methods of using testosterone, please visit my website at www.protealife.com.

78. Margo and Winn, "Testosterone Treatments," 1591–1598.

79. John Kane, Jonathan Middle, and Marion Cawood, "Measurement of Serum Testosterone in Women: What Should We Do?" *Annals of Clinical Biochemistry* 44, no. 1 (2007): 5–15.

80. Frank Z. Stanczyk, "Measurement of Androgens in Women," *Seminars in Reproductive Medicine* 24, no. 2 (April 2006): 78–85.

81. Margo and Winn, "Testosterone Treatments," 1591–1598.

Neurotransmitters

Neurotransmitters require a specialized test. When I run them, I make sure to use a CLIA-accredited lab. CLIA, the Clinical Laboratory Improvement Amendments, are the federal accrediting standards for labs.

The test for neurotransmitters, either a serum test or a morning urine panel, will test for the neurotransmitters we discussed in chapter 6: serotonin, melatonin, and GABA. And the treatment protocol is pretty straightforward. If a neurotransmitter is deficient, it should be treated.

For example, if you present with depression, your doctor should run your serotonin pathway using a basic serotonin panel, which is a very inexpensive but effective lab. Sometimes when you're under high stress, your body turns serotonin into something called kynurenic acid instead of 5-HTP.[82,83] If you have an excess of 5H1AA and a serotonin deficiency, that indicates a B12 folic acid problem. The folic

82. J. Chiappelli et al., "Stress-Induced Increase in Kynurenic Acid as a Potential Biomarker for Patients with Schizophrenia and Distress Intolerance," *JAMA Psychiatry* 71, no. 7 (2014): 761–768, doi:10.1001/jamapsychiatry.2014.243.

83. Hideki Miura et al., "A link between Stress and Depression: Shifts in the Balance between the Kynurenine and Serotonin Pathways of Tryptophan Metabolism and the Etiology and Pathophysiology of Depression," *Stress* 11, no. 3 (2008): 198–209.

acid irregularity causes you to have insufficient serotonin, which is most likely causing your depression.

This section is not meant to be a substitute for professional medical care. It is instead intended to help guide you to your next step.

I spent a considerable amount of time debating what to put into the treatment section of this book. For me, as a physician, it is hard to hold back. I love to discuss the nuances of protocols, with different methods of approaching cases and unique treatment plans that have worked in the past. The problem is that treatments are incredibly dynamic. Research moves quickly, and often we see common treatments give way to newer, more effective ones.

In order to keep this section updated and current, I have provided free digital and downloadable resources at www. protealife.com. There, you will find helpful handouts with the most current protocols in use, along with the cited research to support its clinical value. I have also included talking points to help facilitate a constructive dialog with your care provider.

Combined with understanding the whole picture of your body, these resources can provide the bridge you need to take charge of your health.

How to Find and Communicate with the Right Doctor

A crucial part of treating hormone imbalance is finding a doctor who cares.

The definition of the word *doctor* comes from the Latin word *docēre*, which means "to teach." The role of your physician is to educate you on what's going on inside of your body, to ensure that every decision you make regarding your health is an educated one.

Unfortunately, doctors who work by this definition are hard to find these days.

When most women see a doctor, they expect him or her to just say, "Oh, here's a pill to stop your symptoms," and send them on their way. The doctor prescribes Xanax, Zoloft, pain medication, or stronger birth control. These medications are what these women are supposed to use to manage anxiety, irritability, menstrual pain and irregularity, and other issues related to hormone imbalance.

Most women come in expecting this rote response from their doctor. They're resigned to the fact that most likely no one will offer to sit down with them and deconstruct what the heck is actually going on.

Their health care providers act like they don't care.

I define "caring" as someone sitting down with you and saying, "Let's figure this out together. Let's really get to the bottom of this and understand you, because you're worth that." You deserve a doctor who cares.

If you feel like your doctor doesn't care, it may be time to find a new doctor.

The biggest signs you need to see someone else come down to communication. How does your doctor communicate with you? Does he or she listen to you and then have a back-and-forth discussion about your options? Or is your well-cited research dismissed and tossed aside? Can your doctor cite any statistics or scientific studies he or she mentions? You are not being nitpicky by wanting to know more.

It's important to communicate with your doctor in clear facts as much as possible. Use scientific rationale. If you show your doctor research, he or she is obligated to say, "I don't believe this is correct, *and this is the reason why*. This is the study I'm going to cite." Part of being a good doctor means being a good scientist.

I want you to be able to walk into your doctor's office and say, "This is my body, and I have these symptoms. I would like you to look at these things, because I'm not sure which one is the problem. Once we figure that out, I want you to create a protocol for me to try. Then I want you to test me again in a month, to see if it moves things in the right direction." When you can say this to your doctor and receive a positive response, you know you're in good hands.

If your doctor yells at you, doubts you, makes you feel stupid, or treats you like a nuisance for being proactive about your own health, that doctor is not worthy of you. Finally, if you have a discussion with your doctor using rational facts and he or she still says, "I'm not going to listen to you," you need to find a new doctor.

You deserve to be healthy. You deserve to be cared for. You deserve to be treated with respect.

This is your life. And you are worthy of the best life possible.

Will Work for You

Some people treat doctors like gods. Some think of them as artists or philosophers. Others say that we're like mechanics.

I think you should treat your doctor like he or she is your employee.

I mean it. You need to start looking at me like I'm someone you hired to work for you.

We are so used to hearing doctors tell us, "Just do this." Instead, I want you to start having a relationship with your doctor where you can say, "I don't feel well." And if your doctor doesn't get it right the first time, you come back and say, "I still don't feel well."

When I hear "something doesn't feel right" from my patients, it makes me work even harder to figure out what's going on. That's my job. And I take pride in my work, because I want everyone I see to be healthy and feel happy and sane—not crazy and unheard.

I want you to be happy, too.

And that is absolutely possible. Now that you have all of this information, I want you to move into a brighter future. I'll give you a final few hints about moving in that direction in the next chapter.

Chapter 8

A Beautiful Future

Julie's New Story

Do you remember the story of Julie that I shared with you in chapter 2? Julie was lost and struggling after a lifetime of feeling ignored and dismissed by her doctor.

But it doesn't have to be that way. After Julie learns the same information you have just learned, with a new understanding of her body and her mind, she has a new story. And the earlier she learns, the faster it can begin. It goes like this.

At age thirteen, Julie experiences irregular periods complicated by severe cramping. Julie's mother and father—her health care advocates while she is a minor—seek out a physician experienced in treating young women her age. They find one who first works to discover the cause of hormone problems instead of dismissing her with a prescription for birth control. Her doctor tells Julie that she was right to come in; her symptoms are not normal. He also informs her that these symptoms can be caused by low progesterone, common at her age.

Julie's doctor runs a battery of labs to make sure that nothing more complicated is happening. When the labs confirm his suspicions, he prescribes a course of low-dose natural progesterone. He retests her each month and keeps Julie on this therapy for a few months until she begins to naturally generate her own progesterone. Then she is able to stop taking it because she no longer needs to. Her body makes enough on its own.

When Julie enters college, she does so with a normal level of testosterone because she never took oral contraceptives. She doesn't have the same weight gain that her classmates experience. With normal testosterone levels, Julie's body responds to exercise with healthy muscle development and optimal fat metabolism.

When she has her children, Julie doesn't suffer from postpartum depression. She knows that low progesterone can cause depression, and she is aware of how common it is for a woman to have lowered levels after birth. Her obstetrician follows her case, periodically testing her labs. When she does notice a deficiency, the doctor prescribes natural progesterone to maintain Julie's neurological health.

Julie never needs to take an antidepressant.

After her three children are born and before she goes back to work full time, Julie consults her doctor regarding work-life balance. She and her husband create a healthy schedule that equally distributes the housework as well as the responsibility of parenting. With this balance, she can advance her career and feel fulfilled in her home life.

In her mid-thirties, Julie begins to experience some anxiety. Her physician affirms that this is happening possibly due to diminishing levels of progesterone, common for a woman in her age group. She is early premenopausal, and her body is losing its ability to generate progesterone naturally. Once he confirms this hypothesis, Julie is given a long-term protocol including prescribed progesterone and regular lab work. Her anxiety disappears.

Julie notices some weight gain when she is in her forties. Her physician runs a thorough exam of her thyroid and discovers she has a diminished amount of the active hormone T3. Julie is told this is a normal aspect of aging. Her physician prescribes her a very low dose of natural thyroid. Her weight normalizes within a few months. Julie sleeps well, has a healthy libido, and feels good. More importantly, her body feels *right*.

Now Julie is empowered to change her narrative.

She is ready to take her health into her own hands.

Woman Power

We are at a point in history where women are becoming empowered in ways they never have been before. Health care needs to be an important part of this swing.

If your doctor is not going to empower you, then you must be able to empower yourself. Because when every single woman, as an individual, takes responsibility for her own health, she can create enormous change—both in her individual life and in the lives of those around her.

Your decisions will no longer be in the hands of an "all-knowing" doctor. You will no longer settle for second-level care. Instead, you will understand what is going on in your body, you will know what first-rate health care means, and you will not accept anything less.

Once you take hold of that power, your example will affect all of the other women in your life as well.

When women change, they share their stories with one another. Once you stand up and show other women what it really means to be healthy and whole, they will want to emulate this reality.

I have a wonderful patient named Darla who was at 38 percent body fat when she started seeing me. Within a year and a half, she lowered her body fat to 18 percent. And at forty-eight years of age, she became a fitness model, just to claim her body for herself. But her transformation didn't stop with her.

Darla became a role model.

Even the young women on my staff ask her, "You're how old? And you're competing in fitness competitions?" They see that she has made this change in her late forties. They see that anybody can make this happen—that they can become functional and healthy. And they are inspired.

My practice is living proof of this transformational domino effect. It is entirely referral based, with no advertising whatsoever. I have helped thousands of women change their lives. But it always starts with one—one woman who comes in and receives the empathy, knowledge, and help she needs. Then she refers someone else, inspiring that woman to take charge of her life as well. And this is just in my one little corner of the world.

So you may start out thinking that you are making changes and taking control of your health for yourself. But you don't even know yet the impact you are going to have. You will start a ripple effect in your world, inspiring other women you know to claim health for themselves. Those women will then inspire change in other women.

And the empowerment will spread to the lives of women everywhere, leading to a major swing in women's health.

"The End" Is Just the Beginning

You are never at the end of learning about your health, because you are never at the end of taking care of yourself. And that doesn't stop with the last page of this book.

My hope is that you will take everything you have learned already and make it real in your life. And then I hope you will keep learning.

I have resources available for you to do exactly that.

For more educational materials on anything we've covered in these chapters, you can access my website at www. protealife.com. There, you will be able to find the research cited in this book, along with more information about what may be going on in your body. As I discussed in chapter 7, you can also print handouts to take to your doctors, so you can directly ask them for the help you need.

You are smart, you are capable, and you are worthy of challenging your doctor, to make him or her work even harder. The resources online will arm you with everything you need to do just that.

You can also learn more about all of this in person via my upcoming talks or workshops. Like the online resources, all of this information can be accessed on the website.

Finally, if you're unable to find a doctor who takes you seriously, who works with you and for you to solve the cause of your problem, you can come to see one of the physicians in my practice. I treat people across the country, and you are always welcome.

Your Beautiful Future

You were meant to live a beautiful life.

Thousands of your ancestors have lived, grown, and thrived to make you exactly as you are. You are the pinnacle of humanity right now.

What your body is going through is extraordinary, and when your body swings out of balance, it can be extraordinarily difficult to grapple with the results. But it doesn't have to be that way. You are meant to be healthy. You are meant to be radiant, beautiful, and remarkable.

And you should never settle for anything short of that.

I know it's possible to reclaim your best self, because I've seen it so many times. I have seen women who have had bad experiences—bad marriages, negative environments, poor diets, unbalanced hormones, horrible trauma—and I've seen them reverse it all. I've seen them shine and go on to lead brilliant lives.

I have been lucky enough to play a small part in the empowerment of these women. But my part is limited to being the person who gives you feedback. I can show you what's possible once your life is in balance. I can show you what it takes to get there. But you are the one who decides to embark on the journey to take control of your crazy hormones.

You are the only one who can make the possibility of health into a stunning reality.

When you choose to follow the pathway to a balanced life, you see that it leads to the place where you are supposed to be. A place where you feel happy and complete. A place where you can look in the mirror and love who you see.

You are meant to feel like your best self. You deserve it. Never be afraid to take your health into your own hands.

Then build the beautiful life you imagine. And never look back.

ABOUT THE AUTHOR

Dr. Brendan McCarthy is an internationally recognized expert in hormone replacement therapy. He founded the Protea Medical Center in 2006, where he currently serves as chief medical officer. Dr. McCarthy has helped Protea grow and evolve into a dynamic medical center that helps thousands of patients in the Phoenix Valley and throughout the southwest United States.

We often look at the qualifications of a physician, but choosing a good doctor is about more than just credentials; a good doctor needs to be compassionate and empathetic. Dr. McCarthy has built his practice upon his dedication to each individual patient. He is passionate about educating patients so they are empowered to gain control of their health. Dr. McCarthy also lectures physicians and pharmacists on topics such as weight loss, infertility, hormone replacement therapy, and nutritional therapy.

Dr. McCarthy's hallmark is his unorthodox approach to mental and emotional wellness, as well as its link to hormone balance in women. Through a combination of clinical investigation and blood work, Dr. McCarthy is persistent in his pursuit of possible causes for conditions such as anxiety, depression, PMS, slow metabolism, and more.

Dr. McCarthy spends his free time hiking, swimming, and traveling with his wife, Celeste, and their three children, Liam, Aedan, and Audrey. A three-time Ironman and avid Olympic weightlifter, Dr. McCarthy lives his message of whole-body health, happiness, and well-being.

WHOLE-BODY HEALTH
CAN BE YOURS

Are you ready to feel your best? Dr. McCarthy is dedicated to your success.

He and the staff at Protea Medical Center encourage patients and health care providers to reach out and learn new ways to take control of whole-body health. Dr. McCarthy provides

- In-person speaking engagements for your group or organization
- Small- and large-group physician training in bio-identical hormone replacement therapy
- On-site, one-on-one clinical training at his Arizona facility
- Personalized medical care for out-of-state patients interested in traveling to his clinic

For more information, visit www.ProteaLife.com or call (480) 557-9095.

You can connect with Dr. McCarthy on

- Email: info@ProteaLife.com
- His website: www.ProteaLife.com

Made in the USA
Monee, IL
20 January 2023

25725370R00075